HOW TO
RAISE
A
GENTLEMAN

Other GentleManners™ Books

How to Be a Gentleman
John Bridges

A Gentleman Entertains
John Bridges and Bryan Curtis

As a Gentleman Would Say
John Bridges and Bryan Curtis

A Gentleman Gets Dressed Up
John Bridges and Bryan Curtis

A Gentleman Walks Down the Aisle
John Bridges and Bryan Curtis

Toasts and Tributes
John Bridges and Bryan Curtis

50 Things Every Young Gentleman Should Know
Kay West with John Bridges and Bryan Curtis

50 Things Every Young Lady Should Know
Kay West with John Bridges and Bryan Curtis

How to Be a Lady
Candace Simpson-Giles

As a Lady Would Say
Sheryl Shade

How to Raise a Lady
Kay West

A Lady at the Table
Sheryl Shade with John Bridges and Bryan Curtis

A Gentleman at the Table
John Bridges and Bryan Curtis

A Gentleman Abroad
John Bridges and Bryan Curtis

HOW TO RAISE A GENTLEMAN

REVISED AND EXPANDED

A CIVILIZED GUIDE TO HELPING
YOUR SON THROUGH
HIS UNCIVILIZED CHILDHOOD

KAY WEST

THOMAS NELSON
Since 1798

NASHVILLE   DALLAS   MEXICO CITY   RIO DE JANEIRO

Published in Nashville, Tennessee, by Thomas Nelson. Thomas Nelson is a registered trademark of Thomas Nelson, Inc.

Thomas Nelson, Inc., titles may be purchased in bulk for educational, business, fund-raising, or sales promotional use. For information, please e-mail SpecialMarkets@ThomasNelson.com.

ISBN: 978-1-40160-461-5

The Library of Congress has cataloged the earlier edition as follows:

West, Kay, 1955–
How to raise a gentleman / Kay West.
       p. cm.
ISBN 10: 1-55853-940-9
ISBN 13: 978-1-55853-940-2
1. Child rearing. 2. Etiquette for children and teenagers. 3. Etiquette for boys.
I. Title.
HQ769 .W446 2001
649'.132—dc21
             2001004338

Printed in the United States of America

12 13 14 15 16 WOR 6 5 4 3 2 1

For my parents, who taught me manners; For my children, who taught me parenting; And to RRT, for the rest

CONTENTS

INTRODUCTION

Moments after your newborn son's squalling
entry into the world, he will be weighed,
measured, and take his first test, the APGAR, an
evaluation of his physical condition. A high score is
a relief, but not necessarily reason to download an
application to Harvard or run out and buy a batting
cage.

In this competitive world, parents scrutinize their
son's every move or passing interest for signs that he
might be "gifted" in some field—if his crayon scribble
suggests a superior understanding of proportion and
perspective; if his sturdy frame portends a future
NFL running back; if his skill at assembling Lego
structures predicts a budding architect.

With the goal of identifying and nurturing a
unique talent or special skill, young boys are enrolled
in art classes, signed up for peewee football, and
immersed in technology and accelerated learning

programs. But sometimes in the drive to help our sons succeed, we skip over the one thing that every single boy has the potential to achieve: good manners.

Among the hundreds of expenses that constitute the soaring costs of raising a child from conception to graduation, the development of manners is the least costly. In fact, it is absolutely free. And the bonus is that teaching your son good manners is the one investment you can make with guaranteed returns. He may be trilingual by the time he's in second grade, but if he doesn't say "please" and "thank you" in at least one language, he is at a disadvantage among those who do. He may be able to sketch an impressive self-portrait, but if he doesn't write a thoughtful thank-you note to the family who took him to the beach for a week, he probably won't be asked again. He may have the highest batting average on his Little League team, but if he berates a teammate who strikes out, the coach won't think much of his leadership potential.

Good manners are born from common courtesy and common courtesy is quite simple. Courtesy is based on respect, civility, kindness, and consideration. It is being mindful of others, whether you are in their presence or not. Courtesy walks hand in hand with good manners, and both are the embodiment of the Golden Rule: Do unto others as you would have them do unto you.

Young gentlemen spring forth from any well; blue-blooded breeding does not always lead to blue-ribbon manners. Princes-in-waiting may be more accustomed to fine dining than boys raised on a pig farm, but familiarity with place settings and the proper use of forks is less valuable than kindness and the proper use of "please" and "thank you."

Good manners begin with the assimilation of the examples set for a boy by his parents. *How to Raise a Gentleman* is a book for parents who want to do the right thing but may need a few pointers. This is not a book of formal etiquette but a guide to good manners supported by a commonsense collection of real-life advice, time-tested tips, and lessons learned. Ideally, this instruction manual will prove to be as helpful for parents as it is for sons.

Good manners will open more doors, charm more acquaintances, and make more memorable first impressions than French, art, and golf lessons combined. The basics can be acquired in toddlerhood and, with daily application, will last a lifetime. It is never too soon to begin or too late to catch up.

LEADING THE WAY TO GOOD MANNERS

26 Things to Remember

Use "please," "thank you," and "excuse me."
  Always.

Wait your turn.

Be generous with compliments and stingy with
  criticism.

Listen to your child when he speaks to you, even if
  you've heard it before.

Do not discipline your child in front of others.

Do not correct any child, other than your own, on
  his manners, and always do that privately.

Be clear about what you expect.

Be consistent.

Do not give in to temper tantrums.

Do not lose your temper.

Admit when you are wrong. Offer an apology when you owe one.

Let your child know when a discussion has become a decision.

Words can hurt. Do not hurl them about as weapons.

Respect your child's privacy and boundaries. Knock first.

Do not impose your ideology, and respect those whose ideology differs from your own.

Agree to disagree.

Give credit where credit is due.

Hold the door.

Lend a hand.

Be a good sport.

Be a gracious loser and a generous winner.

Give more than you are asked.

Don't take more than you need.

Leave a place cleaner than you found it.

Do not respond to rudeness with rudeness.

Winning is not the only thing, and nice guys do finish first.

Chapter One

PLEASE, THANK YOU, EXCUSE ME, AND OTHER EARLY SOCIAL INTERVENTIONS

After "Mama" and "Papa," the very next word in your son's vocabulary will likely be "no." In the early stages using the word "no" typically does not indicate rudeness but rather a self-satisfied delight in finding a means to communicate displeasure other than crying, screaming, or squalling. It is also an easier word for tiny mouths to form than the more agreeable and pleasant "yes." As your boy's vocabulary expands, he will begin to communicate his wants and needs. This is the time to introduce the two magic words: "please" and "thank you."

As with most mannerly conduct, the best way to promote its practice is by example. Children want to emulate the adults in their lives and fit in with the rest of the family. If the words "please" and "thank you" are used without exception in your home, your budding young gentleman will follow suit. Using "please" and "thank you" yourself is also an opportunity to reward and promote other courteous behavior. "Thank you for using your fork instead of your fingers." "Please don't leave your shoes in the middle of the floor."

Except in the case of an emergency, encourage the use of the word "please" by not responding to a request until the word is employed. Do not expect a three-year-old to deliver lengthy sentences such as "May I please have a cookie?" but help him see the difference between a request and a demand. "Cookie!" is a demand that grates on the nerves and will go unheeded. "Cookie, please?" is a request so agreeable to the adult ear that it is likely to be met with the cheerful bestowal of the coveted item. (There are exceptions of course: cookies before meals is a no-no in my house, but I try to recognize the mannerly request by saying, "Because that was such a nice way to ask, it's hard to say no, but not before dinner. Maybe afterward.)"

When your son's request is granted, he then responds by saying, "Thank you." Adults should, in turn, respond to this seminal display of civility with a modest expression of approval. A smile or quick hug is fine; rewards are not necessary for behavior that is eventually expected to be a matter of course, with the possible exception of potty training. In that taxing endeavor, the reward system is encouraged. Reserve your applause for accomplishments that deserve it, like an excellent report card, a four-minute mile, or a full scholarship to college.

It is one small but impressive step from "please" and "thank you" to "yes, please" and "no, thank you," but one not to be expected until the child has mastered the former and uses them as habit. By then, "Would you like a cookie?" has two appropriate responses: "Yes, please" or "No, thank you."

The next phrase central to a young man's socially correct lexicon is "excuse me." The opportunities for its use will present themselves again and again:

If a young man inadvertently burps aloud or passes gas in the company of others, the minor offense will be easily forgiven if it is immediately followed by a polite "Excuse me."

• • •

If a young man accidentally jostles another person or steps on toes, the appropriate way to make amends is simply by saying, "Excuse me."

• • •

A young gentleman does not interrupt adults when they are engaged in conversation—in person or on the telephone—but if the conversation is a lengthy one, and he has a pressing need that must be promptly attended to, then he might say, "Excuse me, Daddy. I really need to go to the bathroom now!" An attentive daddy will stop discussing last night's hockey game and attend to his son's request.

• • •

Should a young man need to have something repeated to him because it was unclear or he was unable to hear, he says, "Excuse me?" He does not say, "What?" or even worse, "Huh?"

You Know You Are Raising a Gentleman If . . .

He uses "please," "thank you," and "excuse me" on a consistent basis.

He speaks when spoken to.

He does not point out other children's lack of manners.

When he doesn't understand something, he simply says, "Excuse me?" or "Would you repeat that?"

Parent Pointers

Use "please," "thank you," and "excuse me" in all encounters.

Say "please" when making a request of your son.

Say "thank you" to your son after he fulfills that request.

Say "excuse me" if you must interrupt him, even if it's something as aggravating as a scene-by-scene recounting of a Batman movie.

Occasionally note your son's developing sense of good manners.

Compliment your son's friends on their good manners—but do not reprove them for a lack thereof.

Pass along to other parents what lovely manners their sons have. There is nothing a parent likes to hear more about their son than "Harry has such wonderful manners."

Try This at Home

My sister is convinced that the moment a parent
gets on the phone or goes into the bathroom there
is an alarm that goes off, audible only to children,
that inspires an immediate and pressing need for a
parent's attention. My own experience has proven her
correct. To discourage telephone interruptions from
my son, I simply hold my hand up in front of his little
face like a policeman stopping traffic or turn my back
altogether. Unless it is an emergency, I do not stop my
conversation until its natural conclusion. When in the
bathroom, I lock the door to discourage walk-ins.

Some Good Advice

When I was six years old and apparently quite smug
about my superior manners, I pointed out to a friend
lunching with me that she had not thanked my mother
for her grilled cheese sandwich. My mother called
me to the kitchen and pointed out to me that by
making my friend feel badly, I had exhibited far worse
manners than she. Always remember that the core of
good manners is not steadfast attendance to the rules
of etiquette, but kindness, respect, and consideration
for others.

Chapter Two

YES SIR, NO SIR, AND OTHER REGIONAL DIVIDES

P eople who live in the South often consider a Yankee's typical straightforwardness as discourteous. Conversely, many Yankees take a southerner's love for idle chitchat with complete strangers as an unwelcome and extremely annoying intrusion. Without question there is a perception that Yankees are rude and southerners well mannered. But having lived both north and south of the Mason-Dixon line, I have found plenty of examples of Yankee hospitality and southern chill.

Generally, southerners routinely embellish conversations with elaborate compliments, a practice Yankees consider a waste of time and phony. When I first moved to the South, I was leaving a small market and heard the proprietor say, "Come back soon!" I was stymied. I knew I would never be in again, so I began to explain that I didn't live in the neighborhood and probably wouldn't be back. The cashier looked at me as if I were an alien, which in a sense, I was.

Nowhere are the cultural divides more clearly drawn than in the use of "Sir" and "Ma'am." There is one school of thought that believes children should be taught to use the titles "Sir" and "Ma'am" whenever they interact with an adult. Young men who attend military academies will also be expected to employ this form of address, and its omission can be cause for a strong reprimand.

Otherwise, "Yes, Ma'am" and "No, Sir" are forms of courtesy that are rarely heard in the Northeast or on the west coast. In the South, however, and in parts of the Midwest, such as Kansas and Oklahoma, they are deep-rooted customs.

Growing up in the Northeast, the only opportunity I had to hear children my own age use the words "Yes, Ma'am" and "No, Sir" was when watching *The Waltons*. For the most part, life in the Waltons' home was harmonious. It would have been unthinkable for John-Boy to respond to his mother, Olivia, without saying, "Yes, Ma'am" or "No, Ma'am."

When I moved to the South, I was amazed to find that this habit was not a television fabrication but was standard for many families, though not taught or practiced as frequently or as stringently as it once was.

Teaching your son to use "Sir" and "Ma'am" is a matter of personal taste, with some guidance necessary for its use. If you choose to require it from your son, do it consistently. It is confusing to require the titles for distant members of the family rarely seen but not for Uncle Ted who drops by the house once or twice a week, or to use one practice for close friends of the family and another for professional acquaintances. It is not up to the child to assess the level of the relationship. The measures for the usage of "Ma'am" and "Sir" are quite simple: age and status, with age being the primary consideration. As adults are always older than children, then "Sir" and "Ma'am" are used in conjunction with "Yes," "No," or "Excuse me" whenever your son speaks to an adult, including his parents. This is true even if your twelve-year-old financial whiz kid has accumulated millions in the stock market and could buy and sell every adult in the room. By virtue of their years, they are still his superiors, and he should treat them accordingly.

For some adults the policy governing the use of "Ma'am" and "Sir" is not so grounded in tradition or formalities as it is a means to eliminate such grating responses as "Huh," "Yeah," or "Nah." If your son attends a school where proper deportment is a part of the curriculum, his teachers may require the use of "Sir" and "Ma'am" in the classroom. Even if that is inconsistent with your habits at home, teacher rules always take precedence in the classroom.

You Know You Are Raising
a Gentleman If . . .

He routinely uses "Sir" and "Ma'am" if it is a
practice in your family.

He doesn't remark unkindly on another's accent,
unfamiliarity with English, or regional or
cultural speech patterns.

He does not tell another child that using "ain't" is
bad grammar. It is bad grammar, but it is not up
to your son to point that out.

He follows without hesitation the practices and
rules of conduct when visiting someone else's
home, such as removing shoes before entering or
not feeding the dog from the table.

He does not make disparaging remarks about the
customs or practices of people unlike himself.

Parent Pointers

Use "Sir" and "Ma'am" in appropriate situations if
you require its use from your son.

Do not require the use of "Sir" and "Ma'am" from
anyone other than your own son if other children
are not in the habit of using it.

Do not discourage its use from boys who do, even
if your own son does not. It is not appropriate to
respond to a young man's reply of "Yes, Ma'am"

with a shudder, an admonishment that you are
not his grandmother, and an order not to do it
again.

Deliver a reminder, when needed, in a quiet
and subtle manner. Veteran users of "Sir" and
"Ma'am" report that once mastered, it becomes
a lifelong habit.

Try This at Home

If your son has not yet traveled outside of his
hometown, he may not realize that other people talk
differently than he does and have expressions of
speech unique to their region of the country. If he was
born and raised in Boston, and your college roommate
from Birmingham, Alabama, is coming to visit with
her young son, it would be a good idea to prep him a
little bit on different accents from different parts of
the county so he doesn't laugh if Carter says, "What
are y'all fixin' to do?" Remind your son that it is not
right or polite to make fun of another person's accent,
even if it sounds strange to his ear, and be sure he
understands that to Carter, a Boston brogue sounds
just as odd and unfamiliar as a Southern drawl does to
your son.

Some Good Advice

Before I moved to Nashville, I often traveled there on business. I was amazed by the extravagant displays of Southern hospitality and invitations extended by people I barely knew to come by and see them the next time I was in town. When I moved here and bumped into these same people—people who had given me the impression that they were my future best friends—they were pleasant and welcoming, but none went so far as to extend a formal invitation for dinner. I finally asked a born-and-bred Southern woman why Southern hospitality had suddenly turned so inhospitable. She drawled with a laugh, "Why, Honey, we just love y'all until we find out you're stayin'!" She was being a tad facetious, but I learned not to interpret an unfamiliar culture using only my frame of reference.

Chapter Three

INTRODUCTIONS, GREETINGS, AND LEAVINGS

F irst impressions count, and the great majority of first impressions take place during introductions. More than once we have heard the advisory: you never get another chance to make a first impression.

Young children are often given the benefit of the doubt, and even a terrible introductory meeting can be forgiven if the parent apologizes for his son's refusal to come out from behind his father's legs and take his thumb out of his mouth by explaining that Dylan missed his afternoon nap or hasn't had his dinner.

Even for grown-ups introductions can be tricky to navigate and easy to bumble. For children, particularly young or shy children, they can be extremely uncomfortable. In introducing your son to the practice of polite introductions, always keep his age and level of introversion or extroversion in mind.

Children do have another advantage over grown-ups when meeting someone for the first time: simply by not appearing sullen, young boys can be regarded as cute. A boy who does nothing more than smile and venture a shy "hello" might even be regarded as charming and well mannered. A parent can expect little more than that from their three- to five-year-old. Once a boy enters the school system, where he will encounter more grown-ups and authority figures than before, he should know that a little more is expected of him. And by the time he is approaching double-digit years and his social circle has widened, he should have mastered the basics of responding to and making introductions.

Even the youngest of children can be exposed to the rituals and practices of proper introductions, but a fumbling introduction is better than none at all. It is extremely rude, when in a group of people, to encounter an acquaintance or colleague and not perform some type of introduction. If you have completely forgotten a name, you might forewarn the people you are with and hope that they can help you by introducing themselves first, prompting the one whose name you have forgotten to introduce himself or herself as well. If that doesn't work, you may as well come clean and admit to your malfunctioning memory. If your son sees you practicing this basic form of social inclusion without exception, no matter how awkwardly executed it may be, he will come to see that it is normal and courteous behavior.

Very young boys can and should be introduced but not expected to do anything more than stand quietly while pleasantries are exchanged among the grown-ups. Keep in mind the minimal attention span of a very young boy, and do not expect that he maintain this demeanor while grown-ups discuss a protracted business deal or counsel each other on their midlife crises.

According to traditional etiquette there are three basic rules of introduction. The first two are fairly simple; the third can be more complicated, particularly in modern times when status is dictated by so many particulars. It would behoove parents to know these rituals and practices themselves:

1. A man is always introduced to a lady.
2. A young person is always introduced to an older person.
3. A less important person is always introduced to a more important person.

Fortunately, most of us will never be faced with the possibility of having to introduce Brad Pitt to Beyoncé—who would know? As a man, Brad Pitt should be introduced to Beyoncé, but as a younger person, Beyoncé should be introduced to Brad Pitt. And who's to say who is more important—Brad or Beyoncé? Surely they already know each other, so introductions are not necessary. In all other cases, it is best to remember these simple rules and adhere to them whenever possible.

When introducing a young child to an adult, age takes precedence over gender, so the child should always be introduced to the adult. "Harry, I'd like you to meet Mr. Shaw." "Mr. Shaw, this is my son Harry." A four-year-old boy might be confused or startled by an adult thrusting out a hand to be shaken, and considerate people do not put children in that position. A young boy can simply try his hardest to make eye contact and say "hello".

Anticipating the handshaking formality, parents can rehearse with their son at home. Another "rule" is that an older person always extends his or her hand first to a younger person. So in the event that you have an extreme extrovert on your hands, do advise your outgoing son to wait and follow the adult's lead.

As a boy matures, it is most important to teach him the value of standing up straight, making eye contact, and speaking clearly. Slouching about and looking down at the floor or at an area somewhere over the introductee's shoulder implies that the young man is bored, has something to hide, or has something more important holding his interest. Eye contact is not a staring contest; it only takes two or three seconds, but the impression lasts much longer. (It should be noted that among Native Americans, it is considered rude to make direct eye contact with others.)

When a young man is introduced to a grown-up, he may respond with something simple: "Hello" is always preferred over "Hi" and is certainly better than "Hey" in the Southern vernacular or "Yo" in a Northern one. If the person to whom your son is being introduced continues the conversation with "How are you?" he can say, "Fine, thank you." A helpful lesson to be learned early on is that strangers do not really want to know if your head hurts or you have a toothache, but that "How are you?" is just another form of polite speech.

Boys older than seven or eight are capable of shaking hands, a brief conversation, maintaining eye contact, and speaking clearly and loudly enough for the elderly to hear him. A grown-up might say, "Where do you go to school?" and Aaron answers, "Alexander Hamilton Elementary." "And what grade are you in?" "I'm in fifth grade." "Do you like school?" "Yes, I do."

You may be tempted to answer for your child, particularly if he is slow or hesitant in responding. Resist this temptation, along with the urge to nudge, kick, or pinch him. Allow him to work through this— it's not nearly as bad as public speaking. Later, you might commend him for his mature interaction with your boss.

When the exchange is completed and you are leaving, a younger boy can simply say "good-bye". A boy older than ten can be encouraged to add, "It was nice to meet you."

You Know You Are Raising a Gentleman If . . .

He refers to an adult as Mr. Shaw, Mrs. Shaw, or Ms. Shaw until he is asked to do otherwise.

He is cordial and polite when encountering your friends and acquaintances in social situations.

When introduced to a stranger, he stands and remains standing until he is told to do otherwise.

When he is the common denominator between two or more strangers, he performs introductions as efficiently as possible. He uses the first and last names among peers. If he is introducing a peer to a grown-up, he refers to the grown-up as Mr., Mrs., or Ms. If he normally calls the grown-up only by first name, he introduces him as Jeff Jones.

When introducing members of his family to others, he explains the relationship. "This is my mother, Mrs. Campanis, and my sister, Lindsay Campanis."

He does not shudder in horror or turn his cheek in disgust when an adult relative is determined to hug or kiss him, but simply bears up as best he can. He will be confronted with far more unappealing social situations during his life.

Parent Pointers

Know the basic rules of introductions.

Always make introductions when people in a group do not know one another.

Always include your son in the introductions, but do not require him to do more than he is comfortable doing.

Do not tell your son to kiss or hug someone when it has not been requested.

Try This at Home

Make a game out of performing introductions, enlisting the aid of siblings, spouse, or friends. In one scenario you and your son are in a public place and you run across the librarian from your son's school. Allow your son to make the introductions: "Dad, this is Mrs. Stringfield, the librarian at my school. Mrs. Stringfield, this is my father, Ronnie Griffin."

Pretend you run into one of your employees at a baseball game. "David, this is John Thompson. He works in the graphics department at the office. John, this is my oldest son, David." David responds, "Hello, Mr. Thompson," and offers his hand if Mr. Thompson offers his first. (Do not instruct a child to call you by your first name without consulting the child's parent first. Some parents prefer that their children address all adults with the proper titles.)

Some Good Advice

When I was growing up, I spent at least one weekend a month at my maternal grandparents' house, which I always looked forward to. Even better, my mother's only sister, Donnie, still lived at home, and though she was seven years older than me, she always allowed me to tag along with her and her glamorous teenage girlfriends. The town they lived in was very small, and it seemed that Donnie knew everyone. In addition she was one of the friendliest people I have ever known, and without exception had at least a smile and a "hello" for everyone we came across. Her warm greeting to total strangers was sometimes met with surprise, but the eventual response was almost always a smile and a "hello" in return. I was a fairly shy child, but I absolutely adored my aunt and strove to do everything she did. She taught me early on that it's not so hard to smile and say "hello", and that even the smallest gesture can inspire a big response.

Chapter Four

SHOPPING, OFFICES, AND WAITING ROOMS

W hen child care is unavailable, babies and pre-toddlers are fairly simple to tote about. Put them in a portable car seat, lay them in a carriage, or strap them onto your chest, pack up the diaper bag, and off you go. Rarely will the appearance of your bundle of joy be greeted with anything less than delight, unless he is engaged in one of the following: loud and extended bouts of inconsolable crying, projectile vomiting, or an extremely odiferous diaper mess. A well-mannered parent remedies such situations at once, even if it means retreating to the car or returning home.

Once your boy has taken his first steps, however, he will be much more difficult to confine. As soon as a boy is mobile, he should be taught the basics of good manners if he is to accompany his mother or father out in public. The first step in accomplishing this might be to convey the idea that going along to the dry cleaner, the grocery store, or the bank is not a burden, but an opportunity to spend time together. At least that's how I remember it.

I was the oldest of five children, all born within a space of nine years. My mother was a stay-at-home mom with an endless stream of tasks, and there was little one-on-one time with any of her children. Once a week she did her grocery shopping, and every one of us vied to be the chosen one who would tag along.

My father, in order to support a family of seven, worked one full-time and two part-time jobs, one of which was as a mechanic at a service station. From the time they were about seven years old, my father took my brothers with him to the service station on Saturday afternoons. There, they were expected to do little chores. When not so engaged, they were allowed to sit with the men in the molded plastic chairs that sat in a line outside the entrance to the service station, get a bottle of pop, and listen to man talk. They spoke when spoken to but otherwise kept quiet and gave up their chair if another man needed it while waiting for his car. (Women did not darken the doors of service stations in those days—back when there were full-service stations.)

We felt special just for being allowed to share that time with our parents, and that privilege gave us a sense of responsibility for our behavior. Unlike teenagers, young children want to spend time with their parents, whether sitting down to hear a story, playing Chutes and Ladders, or going along to the bank. Errands might not be as much fun as playing a game, but children must eventually learn that even unpleasant things can be borne with as pleasant a nature as possible.

For quick errands such as banking, going to the post office, short shopping trips, or picking up material at an office, boys do not need to be provided with a diversion, but in all fairness, should be given as accurate an idea as possible of the duration of said errand. Children should never be required to accompany their mothers when shopping for shoes or their fathers when looking at paint colors. You are asking for trouble.

Children should not be expected to endure lengthy waits in a doctor's or dentist's waiting room without some type of diversion. Pediatrician offices usually come equipped with toys and books, but don't count on it. Pre-readers can carry a bag containing a coloring book, some small Matchbox cars, or a self-contained puzzle. Balls of any type are a bad idea anywhere but parks or gymnasiums. Older boys should be encouraged to bring a book, but small, handheld game systems are another option, as long as any annoying sound is turned off.

If you must bring your child to the office with you while you meet with a colleague or complete a task, it is your responsibility to provide your child with something to occupy him, and it is your son's responsibility to remain focused on that task or pastime. Under no circumstances is he to touch things that do not belong to him or to rummage through someone's desk.

When shopping or doing other errands with his parent, a young man should be expected to stay within sight and not run willy-nilly up and down the cereal aisle while his mother or dad is in the dairy department. If the young man cannot control himself in the grocery store, he will have to ride in the cart until he can. This applies to ten-year-olds as well as four-year-olds.

In line at the checkout, a young man does not badger his father for one of the sugary treats displayed at the child's-eye view, though the manufacturers do their best to assure that children will. Make it clear immediately to the young man that badgering will not result in anything favorable, or you leave yourself open to a lifetime of badgering.

In stores, as in offices, children do not touch things that do not belong to them, which includes everything. Even if—or especially if—your child is in a stroller, this notion must be reinforced. I thought my three-year-old son and I were going to be hauled off to jail the afternoon we left a sporting goods store and unbeknownst to me—until we were stopped by the mall security guard—my son had swiped a stainless steel coffee mug, a pricey pair of leather gloves, and a compass-tachometer, all of which were resting in his lap. Thankfully, we were simply asked to return the pilfered goods and make our apologies, and his budding criminal record was expunged.

You Know You Are Raising a Gentleman If . . .

He stays close by the adult on duty in public places. This shows good manners, as it saves the adult from having to raise his voice or chase the child about. It is also a vital safety habit.

In grocery stores and markets, he does not take more than one sample when they are made available.

He accidentally makes a mess in a grocery store and informs a grown-up so that the mess can be cleaned up. He does not need to pick up the mess himself or pay for any broken items.

When forced to accompany his mother or father on a clothing-buying expedition, he never peeks under the dressing room wall to spy on another customer.

He does not mess up someone's desk, rummage through drawers, use a telephone, or log on to someone's computer when at an office. He also asks permission before eating or drinking anything.

He occupies just one seat in the waiting room close by his parent. If the waiting room is crowded and another adult needs a seat, the young gentleman gets up and takes a small, unobtrusive spot on the floor.

In waiting rooms, he does not hog all the books or puzzles but takes just one as he needs it, then returns it to the pile when he is finished.

He uses trash receptacles in public places. A young gentleman does not leave a candy wrapper or used tissue on a chair in a waiting room or on a counter at the post office.

PARENT POINTERS

Do not expect a child to endure a lengthy shopping trip unless it is to a toy or candy store.

Provide a child with diversions if the wait is expected to be a lengthy one.

Give the child an accurate idea of how long the errands will take. Telling a child that the rounds of post office, dry cleaner, bank, and appliance repair store will "just be a few minutes" is misleading at best.

Do not promise a reward at the outset, but if a successful trip is accomplished, offer some small token of appreciation for his good behavior and manners.

Try This at Home

In spite of your best instructions, and your son's best intentions, there is a good chance that sooner or later you and your son may get separated in a mall, department store, movie theater, or market. Practice at home what your child should do if he gets separated from his parent. He should find an employee or security guard, tell that person he is lost, and stay put until his parent is found.

Some Good Advice

No matter how tempting it is not to drag a small child into the post office to buy a book of stamps or the grocery store to get a carton of milk, never leave a child or children in a parked car alone. The possible consequences are not worth the inconvenience. Never leave any child in a running car; a lunge to turn up the radio can disengage a car from the parked position with tragic results.

Chapter Five

PLAYGROUNDS, PLAYDATES, AND PLAYING WELL WITH OTHERS

When my mother was raising her children, there was no such thing as a playdate. Mothers got together in someone's kitchen for coffee at least one morning a week. Naturally, they brought their babies and toddlers along. Babies were held in laps or deposited in playpens while the mothers chitchatted, drank coffee, and ate Danishes and donuts. Toddlers were deposited in a nearby room of the house— probably not even childproofed—or the backyard, where they remained until someone was bitten or pushed down, the coffee ran out, or it was naptime.

Older children—school-age for example—were shooed out of their house to run or bike to their friends' houses, where those mothers shooed them back outside as well. There they remained until they were called home for meals or bed. Life was simpler then.

Today, at-home coffee klatches have been replaced by getting together at coffee shops—minus the kids. Neighborhoods aren't what they used to be, and the world isn't as safe as it once was, or at least seemed at the time. Hence, we have playdates.

When a young man goes to another child's home for a playdate, he does not tote along a toy chest full of his own things, as if expecting that his friend will not have the caliber of amusements and diversions to which he is accustomed. The exception would be if plans have been made to ride tricycles, bicycles, skateboards, or rollerblades; then the visiting boy brings his own equipment. A host does not ride his bike if he cannot provide one for his friend or if his friend did not bring his own.

A young man treats another child's toys as if they were his own, assuming that he is not destructive with his own toys. If a toy is accidentally broken, a young man apologizes and allows the parents to devise a solution, if one is necessary. A good guest follows the rules of the host home when he is visiting. When the playdate is over, visitors help the host clean up.

If a young man is hosting another child in his home, he is prepared to share his toys. If he owns something that would devastate him to lose, put that toy or possession away before the guest arrives. If a toy is accidentally broken, a young man accepts his guest's apology graciously. The host defers to the guest's wishes with regard to play; when a compromise cannot be reached, sometimes it is necessary for a parent to intervene.

A good host occasionally inquires if his guest is thirsty or would like a snack. The host does not correct another child on his manners but may point out that his mother does not allow children's drinks in the living room. Further, a host quickly and emphatically tells his guest that they do not pull their kitty's tail or let the snake out of its terrarium. When he has company, the host does not engage in exclusionary play such as handheld games for one person. A young gentleman helps his friends clean up, but if his guest does not, a gentleman host does not insist.

On playgrounds, whether with children he knows or children he doesn't, a young gentleman doesn't monopolize a swing, and waits in line for his turn on the slide or climbing walls. When it is time to leave, he picks up his things and carries them to the car or on the walk home.

You Know You Are Raising a Gentleman If . . .

He does not invite a friend over for a playdate without first checking with his parents.

He does not invite himself for a playdate.

He does not say dismissive things about another child's toys, home, or electronic equipment.

He does not turn on appliances or open closed doors when he is visiting another home.

He does not announce that he is hungry or ask for something to eat in someone else's home. He may ask politely for a glass of water if he is thirsty.

He does not roam through the house looking for a bathroom, but he asks where it is.

He uses the bathroom with the door closed, and he flushes and washes his hands when finished.

He tells the parent on duty when he doesn't feel well.

He does not leave the host home or yard without telling a grown-up.

He helps smaller children on the playground.

He waits his turn in line for the slide or climbing stations.

He does not spit water on other children when drinking from the water fountain.

When it is time to leave, a young gentleman comes when called and does not run off into the woods or wrap his legs around the fireman's pole and refuse to go.

Parent Pointers

Always make arrangements for a playdate with the other parents, not through the children.

Set a definite time for the playdate, provide a number where you can be reached, and pick your child up when you say you will.

If you have not met the parents of your son's playdate, introduce yourself; do not simply drop your child off in front of the house.

Provide a change of clothing if bathroom accidents are still a possibility.

Always inform the other parent of your child's allergies or idiosyncrasies (e.g., "Neil cannot eat peanuts and is subject to nosebleeds, and here is how it should be handled").

Never send a sick child to another child's home.

Do not allow a sick child to participate in a playgroup.

Share your family's position on appropriate movies, computer play, television, and video games.

Gently enforce your house rules in your car or home (e.g., "We do not use the words 'shut up' and 'stupid' or curse in our house").

Do not correct another child on his or her manners. "What do you say?" will embarrass a child who hasn't been taught to say "please" or "thank you."

Do not punish another child for unacceptable behavior, but you can stop it (e.g., "I cannot allow you to hit Dylan with the stick"). Depending on the extreme nature of the behavior, mention it without recrimination to the child's parent.

Remove your son from the playgroup for inappropriate or unacceptable behavior. Imploring him not to bite rather than placing him in time-out is not sufficient. If the unacceptable behavior continues, skip one of the playgroup sessions until your child can control himself.

Reciprocate an invitation to play at another child's house with an invitation to play at yours.

Try This at Home

Before a playgroup date have a private talk with your child about including everyone in the fun. Ask him to think about how he would feel if he were left out and how sad you would feel for him. Ask him if he would want to be party to hurting another child's feelings. Anticipate what he might do if others in the group want to leave out another child. Help him figure out ways to include everyone.

Some Good Advice

Because his mother and I were friends, I wanted my son to be friends with her son. Unfortunately, the other mother and I did not see what was quite clear to both boys—they had very little in common. My son is very athletic; hers is not. Her son played with action figures; mine loved to build with Legos. Her son was learning chess; mine had no interest.

Every time we visited each other, Harry's behavior became increasingly discourteous and he was spending more time in time-out than playing with Justin. One afternoon when he kicked a ball that hit Justin squarely in his back, I hauled him inside and asked him what he was thinking. He fairly hissed at me, "I am thinking I don't like playing with Justin!" He expressed himself inappropriately, but he had certainly been sending signals for some time that I had ignored. No matter how much you want it to happen, children should never be forced into friendships with children they don't especially like or with whom they have nothing in common. They should be at least polite and cordial, however, when unavoidably forced to spend time with people with whom they share few interests.

Chapter Six

SLEEPOVERS: FRIENDS AND RELATIVES

One of the great measures of independence in your son's life will be his first sleepover. When is he ready? It's easier to say when he is not.

He is not ready to sleep over at a friend's house if he has not mastered the basics of feeding himself, brushing his teeth, washing himself, and dressing himself. Nor is he ready if he isn't sleeping through the night or if he is still having occasional bed-wetting incidents. In general, boys suffer bed-wetting accidents at later ages than girls, so you must be cognizant of this as it relates to courtesy for the host, and your son's self-esteem. If you have the slightest doubt, it is not worth the humiliation your child will suffer waking up in a friend's home on a wet sheet. If your son thinks he is ready, talk to him beforehand about what to do if an accident happens: he should inform the host parent rather than hurriedly make the bed, hide his nightclothes, and hope no one notices. It is up to his friend and the friend's parents to treat him with the compassion he deserves. If it should happen in your home with a visiting child, do not make a big deal of the incident. Assure him that accidents happen to everyone and get him into a clean set of clothes. You should wash his nightclothes along with the sheets and divert the children's attention as quickly and cheerfully as possible to something else: a special breakfast, Saturday morning cartoons, or outside play. Have a private, thoughtful, and firm talk with your own child at the earliest opportunity to be sure he understands that it was an accident, that his friend probably feels embarrassed, and that it is something that is to remain completely private and not to be spoken of again. Invite that child over again soon to let him know that he is still welcome in your home.

When your son is ready for a sleepover at a friend's house, he packs a backpack with the basics: nightclothes, clean underwear, a change of clean clothes, toothbrush, toothpaste, hairbrush, any medications he is required to take, a sleep toy if he uses one (e.g., stuffed animal or blanket), and in some cases, a pillow and sleeping bag. He may also bring a book and one or two small toys, but not his entire plastic animal kingdom.

A young gentleman follows his host's bedtime rules and does not whine that he is always allowed to stay up until midnight on weekends when he is at home. The host parent leaves some type of night-light on that can guide the child to a bathroom should he wake up in the middle of the night. A child's parents warn the host parents if their child is in the habit of falling out of bed or sleepwalking.

A young gentleman also follows the host house rules when he gets up in the morning. My son will sleep as late as eight o'clock on weekend mornings, but his friend Aaron routinely wakes up at the first light of dawn. One Saturday morning I peeked in around 6:30, and there was Aaron sitting quietly in bed in the dark, a flashlight on his book as Harry snored away in the other bed. I wanted to give him a hug but I didn't want to wake up my son.

If a guest wants to go home, do not make him feel ashamed of being homesick. Likewise, if your child is tentative about spending the night away, assure him that he may call you if necessary.

The first time Harry had a sleepovers planned with a friend, I got emotional as I packed his little bag, drove him over to his friend's house, and waved bye-bye to his rapidly disappearing back as he raced off to play, completely thrilled at the idea of spending a night away from Mom. I didn't hear a peep again until the next day when his friend's dad brought him home all smiles and full of stories about his great adventure. And that's a good thing. Logically I knew that his independence was a healthy sign of his self-confidence and security. In my sentimental mother's eye, however, I was already seeing him loading up his car and heading off to college without a backward glance. Hopefully, when that day arrives, he will do it with the same sense of adventure and confidence that he took with him on his first sleepover.

YOU KNOW YOU ARE RAISING A GENTLEMAN IF . . .

He keeps his belongings in the proper places and cleans up his space.

He leaves the bathroom as he found it—seat down, water off, towels hung up.

He does not touch or use things that do not belong to him.

He conforms to house rules and schedules.

He informs his hosts immediately if he has an accident of any kind.

He shows a guest around the house, and lets him know where the bathroom, telephone, and exits are located.

He asks his guest what he would like to do.

He does not make fun of his guest if he has an accident, sleeps with a "blankie", still sucks his thumb, or suffers a sudden bout of homesickness and needs to call his mother.

He thanks his host for having him or thanks his guest for coming.

Parent Pointers

Make sure your guests know where the bathroom, your bedroom, and all exits are, but remind them not to leave the house without letting you know.

Have phone numbers of the guest's parents and their whereabouts for the evening.

Share your child's physician's name and insurance carrier, as well as hospital preference, in the unlikely event of an extreme emergency and you cannot be reached.

Share your child's allergies or medical conditions (e.g., the proper use of an inhaler if your child has asthma).

Inform the host of any sleeping problems your child might have, such as: sleepwalking, restlessness, early rising.

Let the host know that if your child suffers an inconsolable bout of homesickness, you are available by phone or to pick him up, no matter the hour.

A divorced parent does not have the person he or she is dating spend the night when the children are at home. Period. Call me rigid and old-fashioned. I don't care.

Try This at Home

The first time my son had a friend spend the night, the friend decided right around bedtime that he needed to go home. He didn't seem too upset, just a little apprehensive about going to sleep in a strange bed. I told him that would be fine if that was what he wanted and asked him if he would like me to call his parents. I spoke to them first and assured them he wasn't hysterical but just seemed unsure. I asked them what his normal bedtime routine was, and they told me that one of them usually got into bed with him and read a story before turning out the light. I said that was exactly what we did, and that I would do that if he decided to stay. They talked to their son, and whatever they said reassured him. When he got off the phone, I told him that Harry always liked me to read him a story in bed and asked if that would be okay with him. We let him pick out a book, and all three of us got into bed and read Dr. Seuss's *Oh, the Places You'll Go*. I turned on the night-light, turned off the overhead light, told them goodnight, and went downstairs. When I went back to check on them ten minutes later, they were both sawing logs. The next morning my son's guest felt like a million bucks for sticking out his first night away from home, and was doubly excited when we made a celebratory trip to Krispy Kreme Donuts.

Some Good Advice

There are all kinds of first sleepovers. While most of us think of them as exciting occasions when our children visit friends or relatives, when parents are divorcing sleepovers can be traumatic. Until my ex-husband, our children, and I attended a course called "Children Facing Divorce," I didn't know the exact nature of the fears my children experienced the first few months they spent the night at their father's new home. As it turned out, they were deeply concerned about what I would do while they were gone, how lonely I might be, and if I were safe at home alone.

If you are facing this situation, discuss this in advance with your children. Tell them that you will miss them, but that you have plans and that you know they will have a great time with their other parent. Speaking from personal experience, I suggest making plans to have some friends over for a casual dinner to help you through those first few times.

Chapter Seven

PARTY MANNERS

I f you thought your social calendar was full before, you will be absolutely agog at what happens once you have children. In addition to your own engagements, your mailbox will soon be brimming with invitations addressed to your child, who hardly seems old enough to be getting his own mail. Most will be of the birthday party ilk, but you will also soon be subject to a stream of summons to an array of family-friendly gatherings and countless opportunities to celebrate children.

One family I know invited sixteen children—and their respective thirty-two parents—to their little boy's first birthday party. It was not a pretty sight.

Dressed in their finest party clothes, the children were cute—for five minutes. Then one started crying, setting off a horrific chain reaction. Many were teething and drooling like St. Bernards. Most were in the first stages of walking, tottering precariously about the room until falling over and bopping their heads.

The parents had engaged a clown who succeeded in terrifying all sixteen children, particularly the birthday boy. The present-opening ceremony went on and on, with not a single child, including Prince Charming, paying one whit of attention. Finally, it was time for the birthday cake. As his parents urged him to blow out the candles and a dozen cameras flashed simultaneously in the poor child's eyes, he chose that very moment to loudly and unmistakably defecate. Whose crazy idea was this anyway?

I am of the opinion that with the exception of immediate family gatherings, children don't need and certainly don't expect big birthday parties until they are at least three years old. Until then, they won't remember a thing anyway. It is a bit unrealistic to expect good party manners from your child until he is about five years old, which is about the youngest age parents can drop their son off at a birthday party and not be expected to stay. (Do not drop a child off without going into the party location and checking in with the parents.)

When your child receives an invitation to a birthday party, it is your responsibility to RSVP promptly. A young gentleman arrives promptly at the party or prearranges a late arrival if a soccer or baseball game conflicts. Once a child accepts an invitation to one party, he cannot reject that offer for another.

On arrival a young gentleman finds the guest of honor and wishes him a happy birthday. Unless he has some physical restrictions that prevent him from doing so, he participates in all party activities. The party is for the birthday child, and by accepting the invitation to the party he has made a tacit agreement to be a cheerful guest.

A young gentleman does not thrust his present in the birthday boy's face, nor does he make disparaging comments about the other gifts. When the cake is presented, he does not shove other boys out of his way to sit beside the birthday boy but takes the first available seat at the table. A guest does not assist in blowing out the candles unless it is requested, and he does not ask for a bigger slice of cake or the piece with the special décor.

When the party is over, he again wishes the guest of honor a happy birthday and thanks him and the parents for being invited.

A birthday boy should assist with the planning of his own party as long as he has realistic expectations. Many parents use the formula of one guest per each year of the child's age; a five-year-old can invite five friends, a ten-year-old can ask ten.

When his guests arrive, the birthday boy greets everyone and makes them all feel welcome. When opening his presents, the guest of honor acknowledges the giver, shows the opened gift to the audience, and offers sincere thanks. He never says, "I don't play with Legos anymore," even if that is true, and he never asks how much a gift cost.

Besides birthday parties, there will be other

opportunities for boys to attend family-inclusive parties from Christmas to the Fourth of July to joyous celebrations such as weddings.

If children are invited to the wedding and reception, it will be noted on the invitation. In most cases boys can wear what they would wear to church or temple. If there is a receiving line, boys can accompany their parents and just say "hello". Children younger than six should not be permitted to carry their plates through the buffet line, but can point out what they would like. Boys six and older can carry their own plates but should not treat a privately funded buffet like an all-you-can-eat breakfast bar.

When people are serving and seating themselves, it is not necessary for a young man to wait for everyone to be seated until he eats. He should not take his used plate back to the buffet for a second helping.

When toasts are offered, he may either remain in his seat or stand with the rest of the guests. If there is dancing, a young man should dance with his mother or grandmother, if they so desire. A young gentleman is under no obligation to ask girls his age to dance, but if he chooses to sit out that portion of the celebration, he does not snicker and make fun of those who participate.

In private homes where seating is at a minimum, a young gentleman does not take a chair when it would prevent an adult from sitting. Instead, he finds a spot on the floor as long as it is not in a walking path or on the middle of a step on a staircase.

A friend of mine passed along her annual Easter egg hunt to us eight years ago when her own children got a little old for the Easter Bunny. It is a very casual affair with about seventy-five children and fifty adults. The children play in the yard, then hunt for the eggs, then everyone spreads blankets on the lawn and collects a plate of food from the buffet.

While the guest list has remained consistent from year to year, as my children have gotten older they have typically invited several new friends. They know it is their responsibility to make sure everyone is included in the fun, and that they will get the evil eye from their mother if even one child is spotted alone or not picked for a spot on one of the kickball teams. It must be working! After the party this year, a first-year Easter egg hunt mother sought me out to tell me how lovely my son had been to her three children, introducing them to the other kids, making sure they were included in the game, giving them egg-hunting tips, and making a place for them on his blanket. I made a mental note to go back to the store and get a jumbo chocolate bunny.

YOU KNOW YOU ARE RAISING A GENTLEMAN IF . . .

He does not talk about a party he is having, or was invited to, in front of other children who are not invited.

He does not go on and on about a party he has

attended or given in front of people who were not there.

He greets and bids farewell to the guest of honor, and thanks his host for including him. He does the same to the guest of honor's parents.

He greets, bids farewell to, and thanks his guests for coming.

He never tries to steal the spotlight at another boy's birthday party.

He does not ask for more of anything—drinks, pizza, cake, or arcade tokens—unless it is offered.

He never says, "I already have this," when opening a present.

He does not screw up his face and say, "Gross, no way!" if his mother, or grandmother, should ask him to briefly sway across the dance floor with her at a wedding. Mothers and grandmothers get sentimental at these affairs.

When and if a young lady is so bold as to ask him to dance, and he would rather undergo a root canal than embarrass himself in front of a hundred people, he still accepts and endures.

Parent Pointers

Send party invitations in the mail or by e-mail if necessary, but do not rely on your son to extend verbal invitations.

Remind your son not to talk about his own party, or a friend's party, in front of other children.

If a soccer game or swim meet will delay your son's arrival at a birthday party by more than thirty minutes, be sure that a late arrival is all right with the hosts. If the delay would be longer than sixty minutes, decline the invitation.

Keep track of who gave which gift so that mention may be made in the thank-you notes.

Be on time to pick children up after the party is over. Inform the hosting parents that you are taking your child.

Do not send extra money with your son to a birthday party held in any place with video games, air hockey, or foosball. It would not do for your son to be playing skeeball while everyone else is being herded into the movie theater.

Be clear about rules of the buffet table. Whatever

he puts on his plate, he is expected to eat. One
dessert, not three.

In hosting, let your son participate as much as
possible in the planning, execution, and cleanup
of the party.

Suggest ways that your son can be sure everyone
is included, particularly children who don't
know other children.

Try This at Home

Here's a possible birthday party scenario with the
potential for hurt feelings that you can discuss
beforehand. Your son opens a gift, and it is something
he already has. He does not mention this but just says
"thank you". If it cannot be returned after the party, he
can give it to a sibling or a charity. If at the same party
he opens a duplicate gift, he just says "thank you" and
moves on.

Some Good Advice

At the beginning of the school year, my son's kinder-garten teacher sent home a list of dos and don'ts for parents. The most thoughtful one was not to send birthday party invitations to school with your child in the interest of saving postage or time unless the entire class is invited. As you will find out, notes sent home with a child, unless in an official school folder, will often remain crumpled up at the bottom of his or her backpack for months. More importantly, the children not invited might suffer serious feelings of rejection, and it can put your own child in an awkward situation if a left-out child asks why he or she was not invited.

Chapter Eight

DINING IN AND OUT

Teaching a child to self-feed is a messy undertaking to say the least. If you thought you had a hard time getting a little bowl of chocolate pudding into his mouth, just wait until he is in control of the spoon. But the only way he will learn is by letting him do it himself.

On those first, cutlery-free attempts, your son's face, hair, ears, hands, clothes, your clothes, the dog, the floor, and everything else within a five-foot radius of him will be covered with whatever he is attempting to get from the high-chair tray to his mouth: chicken fingers, orange slices, cheerios, watermelon pieces, and most adorably, his first birthday cake.

Eventually, with much patience and practice, your child will develop a working relationship with a fork and spoon.

Every young gentleman, as soon as he is able to reach a sink, even if it requires the aid of a stepping stool, washes his hands before coming to the table.

Once he is at the table, seated on a chair or booster seat, the simplest things go a long way toward fostering pleasant dining experiences. Even a young gentleman can be taught not to play with his food, not to chew with his mouth open, not to talk with his mouth full, and to keep his elbows off the table. If parents insist on these common courtesies with consistent reinforcement, they need not fear boorish behavior from their son when the family has company over, dines out, or when their son has dinner at a friend's house.

The assimilation of more advanced skills comes next. The napkin is not intended for use as a paper airplane, a hat, a mask, or a place to deposit chewing gum (always dispose of chewing gum before coming to the table). A young gentleman places his napkin on his lap after being seated and uses it to wipe his mouth and fingers during and after the meal.

No matter how utterly famished he is, a young gentleman waits until everyone is seated before digging into his food. In homes where grace is said, eating begins after giving thanks for the food.

If a young gentleman desires something that is out of his reach, he does not do the boardinghouse reach. Instead he asks: "May I have the butter, please?" or "Please pass the gravy."

A young gentleman who has mastered knife skills to the extent of cutting his own meat or buttering his own biscuits, places the dirty knife on his plate when not in use, not on the table.

A young gentleman must always remember that unless the meal is brought to his front door by a person wearing a uniform, is delivered via a drive-through window, or comes out of plastic or Styrofoam containers, someone in the house has gone to some degree of effort to create a nutritious and delicious meal. A young gentleman does not sit down at the table, look at his plate, and say, "Eeeeew, what's this?"

All parents—even the most sophisticated gourmands—will discover that young taste buds are narrowly defined, and for some time will only respond favorably to foods that can be covered with ketchup, syrup, or melted cheese. Over time this will change as they continue to be exposed to new foods. My son hated spinach, broccoli, and peas until he turned six or seven; now he can't get enough. I do not adhere to the policy of making children eat things they don't like. Children have very distinct likes and dislikes predicated on everything from color to texture. Making him eat something he hates might result in him not trying it again when he's an adult and might actually like the offensive food item.

A young gentleman does not gobble his food as if it was his last meal, but he maintains a good pace by observing his fellow diners. When a young gentleman is finished eating, he asks to be excused before leaving the table.

Dining out with children in full-service restaurants is always an adventure and one for which parents should be sure they are ready. While many diners greet the arrival of children in a restaurant as eagerly as they would a swarm of mosquitoes, the fact of the matter is that children have every right to dine at family-friendly restaurants. Their fellow diners also have every right to expect those children to behave and not to interfere with their neighbors' dining enjoyment. Restaurants that employ maître d's, sommeliers, and Riedel stemware are probably not suitable for children.

When dining out, the same basic rules of the home apply, but even more so. Because there are other people about, a young gentleman does not raise his voice at the table. He has good posture and does not loll about at the buffet table. Unlike at home, where he is called to dinner when it is ready, in a restaurant there is always a wait for food. Many family restaurants provide crayons, place mats, and small games to help children pass the interminable fifteen minutes of downtime, but parents should also be prepared with even something as simple as a small pad of paper.

By the time a young man attends his first formal dinner in an upscale restaurant, at a party, or in a home, he should know the basic rules of bread plates, silverware, and passing:

- The bread plate is the smaller one to the left above the forks. (The salad plate is larger, and also to the left of the place setting or on top of the dinner plate.) Your beverage glass is to the right of your plate.

- A young gentleman takes one piece of bread from a basket without fingering the others, then he passes the basket along to the right. Likewise, he takes one pat of butter from the butter dish (with a butter knife if one is provided), and then passes the butter plate to the right.

- The silverware farthest away from the plate is used first. When a course is completed, a young man puts his used silverware on the plate.

- When serving dishes are being passed family-style, you pass the dishes to the right.

You Know You Are Raising a Gentleman If . . .

He washes his hands before coming to the table.

He comes to the table properly attired.

He removes his cap when he sits down to eat at a table in a home or restaurant.

He keeps all four legs of his chair on the floor.

He does not reach across his dining companions for the salt and pepper shakers.

He does not take the last helping of potatoes or the last roll from the basket without offering it to the table.

He does not eat before the others begin, before his host or hostess is seated, or before the blessing.

He asks to be excused from the table to go to the restroom or when he has finished eating.

He does not ask "What's for dessert?" while everyone is still eating the salad.

When dining out in a restaurant, he does not get up from the table and wander about, nor does he create bizarre and potentially explosive concoctions from the condiments on the table.

He treats the server cordially and with respect, saying "Thank you," when his meal is delivered.

Parent Pointers

Teach by example and always, even during the most casual meals, follow basic dining etiquette.

Do not ask children or guests to say the blessing unless you know they are comfortable with it.

Do not force children to eat what they don't like but encourage them to take a taste.

Never argue at the dinner table. If you are having a squabble, put it on hold during the meal.

Do not watch television during dinner.

If the home phone rings during a dinner, let the call go to voice mail and return it later.

Do not talk on your cell phone at a table in a restaurant. If an emergency occurs, get up from the table and go outside to take the call.

Treat servers and professional help with respect. If the meal or service is not satisfactory, ask to see a manager and make your complaints discreetly.

Always compliment and thank the host or hostess when invited to dine in another's home.

TRY THIS AT HOME

If a parent spends time and effort cooking a meal, the worst thing a young gentleman can do is greet the serving of the meal with one of the following: "Eeeew," "Gross," "Yuck," or "What's that?" A young man should not be surprised if his mother picks up his plate, throws its contents down the sink, and shrieks at him to go to his room for the rest of the night.

That might be a tad extreme and not exactly setting a teachable example, so try this instead. Pick up the crooked little coffee mug your son made for you with his own two little hands last Mother's Day. No doubt he will remember the tears that sprang to your eyes and the huge fuss that rewarded its presentation. Ask him how he would have felt had you opened his gift and said, "Eeeeew, what's this?" Explain to him that the beauty of the coffee mug is immensely enhanced by the fact that he made it just for you, because you are his mother, and he loves you. Tell him you do not expect applause when you set a meal on the table, but that it hurts your feelings when he recoils as if you had set a plate of cow manure before him. I bet he gets the message.

SOME GOOD ADVICE

Do not force a child to eat something he hates. My mother, a child of the Depression, believed you should eat whatever was set before you—all of it. This was terribly painful for my little sister, who hated everything that had ever had any contact with soil. Long after everyone else had left the table, poor Carolyn would be sitting there, forcing down the last of her peas and carrots, green beans, and boiled cabbage. One night just as she finished choking down the last mouthful of pureed butternut squash, her dire warnings to my mother were fulfilled. Every bit of squash and everything else she had eaten that day came back up all over her plate, the table, the floor, and Carolyn. It was disgusting, but dramatic enough that from then on, we were no longer required to eat things we truly loathed.

Chapter Nine

CULTURAL AFFAIRS: THE THEATER, MOVIES, SPORTS, MUSEUMS, AND LIBRARIES

W hen your children are very small, cultural events will likely be limited to movie theaters showing sixty-minute animated films, story hours in the children's section of bookstores and public libraries, and the occasional puppet show. Once they are mobile and talking, parents must enforce self-control from their youngsters during a performance, no matter how many unruly heathens are running about unfettered. It is not up to you to police other children, though you can certainly try to lead by example. As they get older, they will have occasion to frequent performances, events, and cultural institutions that require more refined manners and a more mature level of behavior.

The first step in promoting good audience manners is making certain a boy is old enough to enjoy the experience or at least endure it with a minimum of fidgeting. You will not foster a love of the ballet by dragging along a reluctant young man who would rather spend an hour at the orthodontist than sit through *The Nutcracker*. In fact, it may do more harm than good. Good behavior comes naturally when a child is enchanted by what is taking place before him. A young gentleman may never develop a love for the opera, but he is expected to exhibit a healthy respect for the efforts and skills of the artists and craftspeople behind the production. Anyone can bear anything for three hours, and it is good training for the future when he will have to endure far worse.

Children's theater is a wonderful introduction to the stage. The productions are lively, often including audience participation, and most importantly, they are shorter than adult theater. Alfresco performances, such as Shakespeare in the Park, are other fine ways to ease children into the pleasures of the play. If the dialogue onstage sails over their heads, a bored young gentleman can occupy himself by lying on his back and gazing at the stars.

Once it has been determined that a child is old enough to sit relatively still for two to three hours and plans are made to attend a play, the opera, a symphony concert, or the ballet, a young gentleman should be told what to expect and what is expected of him.

For a live production of any type, members of the audience arrive on time in order to be seated before the performance begins. It is exceedingly rude to come in after the curtain has risen. If they are tardy, they must wait quietly in the back of the theater until an usher finds the opportunity to seat them. A young gentleman visits the water fountain and restroom before being seated. If his seat is in the center of the row and others are already seated, he says "excuse me" as he approaches and allows them to stand to let him pass or shift their knees out of his way, in which case he must be very conscious of toes. He passes facing them, squeezing his bottom against the seats in the other row. If he is already seated and someone needs to move past him, he should tuck his feet under his chair and make sure the floor is clear in front of him.

Typically, food and beverages are not permitted in performance halls; a young gentleman should discard his chewing gum before entering the theater lest he unconsciously start blowing bubbles. During intermission, he may go to the lobby with his parents or guardian, and enjoy a refreshment if it is offered to him.

A young gentleman does not talk during the performance. If he must ask a question, he whispers into the ear of his mother or father. He does not emit extravagant and dramatic sighs of ennui, and he covers his mouth when he yawns. He does not flip loudly through the program or use it as a fan; wiggle in his seat or swing his legs and kick the seat in front of him; stand up and move about. He follows the lead of the adults in knowing when to applaud or stand for an ovation. He does not place his fingers in his mouth and emit an ear-shattering whistle, no matter how much he loved the aria.

Attending a movie is a far more casual outing than a ballet or opera, but the most basic rules of courtesy, involving unnecessary talking and standing still apply. If he has seen the movie before but his companions have not, he does not tell them the end or announce just before a crucial scene: "Ooooo, watch him fall off the side of the cliff!" A young gentleman does not throw Raisinettes at his classmate sitting two rows in front of him, stick his hand in someone else's popcorn bucket without invitation, suck on a straw or crunch ice loudly, or rest his food and drink in the row where he might inadvertently kick it over and send a river of Dr. Pepper down to the front of the theater. If a young gentleman has set his food on the floor in front of him, and someone passing down the aisle knocks it over, he does not berate that person. When the movie is over, a young gentleman picks up his trash and deposits it in the garbage can located by the door of the theater.

Attending a sporting event is a great opportunity to admire highly skilled athletes, professional or otherwise. For many men, it also seems to be a natural opportunity to release one's frustrations and backed-up testosterone. Witness the popularity of professional wrestling. The judgment of parents who take young boys to such spectacles of boorish, violent, and sexist behavior is curious indeed, and one assumes they are not there to learn gentlemanly behavior. Most other sports, while not as stringent in their rules of conduct as the ballet, do require some courtesy peculiar to that sport.

A young gentleman gets to his seat without disturbing fellow spectators, being careful not to hit anyone in the eye with a foam-rubber tomahawk or knock over an eight-dollar beer. He keeps his belongings in his lap or under his seat, including binoculars, baseball gloves, pennants, and banners with which he hopes to attract the eye of the television cameras. He stands for the singing of the national anthem, always removing his hat. Once the game begins, he sits and remains seated unless a spectacular play occurs, and everyone stands for a better look, or during baseball's seventh-inning stretch. In other sports it is fine to stand, stretch, and move about between quarters or periods. With respect to fellow spectators, a young gentleman does not get up to go to the restroom or concession stand or try to return to his seat during play but waits for a natural break in the action. A young gentleman keeps his food in his lap while he is eating and his beverage in his hand or the cup holder. He does not scatter the remnants of his food and beverage about him—no one wants to step into a pile of leftover nachos—but scoots them under the seat until he can deposit them in a garbage can.

In spite of the behavior of many grown men, buying a ticket to a sporting event does not entitle a young man to scream insults at the players or the opposite team. Likewise, the common practice of cheering on hockey players as they pummel one another mid-ice is disturbing.

When visiting a library, a young gentleman follows the traditional rules of quiet respect for others and a certain reverence for the institution itself. In museums other than those geared specifically to small children, he moves quietly and calmly from room to room in the normal flow of traffic. He stands far enough back from the exhibit to allow others to see. He does not read the descriptions of the pieces aloud unless he is assisting a nonreader, in which case he should do it as quietly as possible. He never touches museum pieces. He does not lie down upon the benches for a quick snooze, no matter how bored he may be.

You Know You Are Raising a Gentleman If . . .

He removes his hat during a performance in a theater without being told to do so.

He disposes of his chewing gum before a live performance.

He removes his ball cap during the playing of the national anthem.

He doesn't cheer when a member of an opposing team is hurt, but applauds when the downed player walks off or is assisted off the field.

He does not boo his own team, no matter how inept their play or how many times they have broken his heart.

He does not say bad things to or about spectators who are rooting for the other team, and does not gloat if his team wins.

He does not knock anyone over while racing to get a ball hit into the stands, or grapple fiercely with others over T-shirt or candy-bar giveaways.

He sits in his seat on his bottom, not on his knees or feet or perched on the armrest, so as not to block the view of those behind him.

He does not make untoward remarks—"That's stupid. I could have painted that!"—about the art he is viewing in a museum or gallery. The audio tour of the exhibit might be enthusiastically received by children accustomed to headphones and ear buds.

He only takes the books he can read during a visit to the library and then takes them to the book cart when he is done.

He takes turns on the computers at the library.

Parent Pointers

Do not force cultural expeditions on your son until he is ready to sit still for the duration.

Educate your son about the respect due performers and fellow audience members.

Before entering a theater, turn your beepers and cell phones to vibrate or leave them in the car.

Make sure bathroom needs are attended to before being seated, and check to be sure chewing gum has been disposed of properly.

Lead the way to the seat.

Carry a cough drop or throat lozenge in case the need arises. If an uncontrollable coughing fit begins, leave the seats for the lobby as unobtrusively and quickly as possible.

Take out of the theater what you brought into the theater.

Never take small children to movies that are clearly intended for adults, whether by virtue of their rating or the sophistication of their content. If you cannot retain a babysitter, wait for another night or enjoy the DVD in the comfort and privacy of your own home.

Do not get into an argument with another audience member over his bad behavior or a spectator at a sporting event for smoking or being intoxicated. Inform an usher and he or she will take care of it.

Exhibit good sportsmanship at sporting events, resisting the urge to point out the shortstop's shortcomings, boo bad plays, get into an argument with a fan of the opposing team, or enjoy too much beer.

Be aware of and versed in the more stringent spectator etiquette of golf and tennis.

Try This at Home

Before attending a play, an opera, or a symphony concert with your son, spend a few moments at home discussing the plot or the composer. Give him a brief outline of the play or the story behind the opera (particularly if it will be sung in another language), the sections of the orchestra, and the conductor's job. A little bit of education opens a window, and an informed viewer or listener is a more interested one.

Before going to a sporting event, read the sports pages together and check where the teams are in the standings, identify each team's key players and any special history between the opponents.

Some Good Advice

When taking a young gentleman to the theater for the first time, you might want to commit to just one-half of the event. That way the boy knows that if he hates it, he can leave at intermission, but if everything is going well, he can stay for the remainder of the performance. Chances are, he'll want to stay to see how things turn out.

Expose your son to museums in small, graduated doses. Do not force a child or young man to endure hours of European portraiture or Early American farming implements.

Chapter Ten

TRAVELING MANNERS

Just a few generations ago, families nearly always traveled together by automobile. As long as the eventual destination was reachable by some combination of blacktop, gravel, and dirt road, then a car was the way to go.

Hidden from the view of anyone outside of the immediate family, packed in the backseat of the car, children were free—as free as their parents allowed them—to be as obnoxious and unruly as anyone would be after four hours in a confined space. In my personal experience, this bad behavior included everything from pinching, poking, punching, and name-calling to what my mother was convinced was deliberate car sickness just to get my father to pull over and let us out. As my mother carried all food and beverage necessities onboard, the only reason to stop was for gas. Until then, we were expected to "hold it."

On one memorable trip my vows of pending and disastrous car sickness went unheeded right up until the moment I leaned over and threw up all over my little sister, who was seated in the middle of the front seat between my parents. After that incident we made fairly regular stops en route, once every two or three hours anyway. It was during one of those stops that we somehow forgot my brother. Five kids got out of the car, and four kids got back in. We were a good half hour down the road before someone noticed Jimmy wasn't in the car, though for a few minutes more, my mother was convinced he was hiding under the beach towels. When we got back to the rest stop, there was my brother, sitting on a high stool behind the information counter like a king on a throne, wearing the highway patrolman's hat, drinking a soda, and eating a candy bar. The rest of us were insanely jealous, which made my mother all the more vigilant during rest stops, determined that no one would get away with a stunt like that again.

The skyrocketing cost of gasoline, coinciding with Americans' fundamental desire to do everything faster, changed all that. I was nineteen the first time I got on an airplane; my children both reached that milestone before their first birthdays. Before I had children of my own, I greeted the sight of a mother carrying a baby or hauling children down the aisle of a plane with the same dread that I would have if she had been toting a bucket of snakes.

The trials and tribulations of motherhood have

since imbued me with unshakable compassion for all parents traveling with small children, but not so much that I would patiently tolerate rude behavior from a child or inattentive or indifferent supervision from an attending adult. In such confined space it is crucial that parents strictly enforce courteous behavior from their children.

The advent of more affordable airfare had the unfortunate side effect of introducing a more casual approach to air travel. I am not lobbying for a return to the days of suit and tie, hats, and gloves, but I would sooner sit three hours beside a screaming, wailing infant than three minutes beside a hirsute man in shorts, sandals, and a tank top who has mistaken his powerful body odor for irresistible pheromones that will result in a date with the cute blonde flight attendant. If a young man is dressed as if he is going to the beach, he will likely act as though he were at the beach. When a young gentleman travels by plane, he dresses neatly in school clothes.

A young gentleman follows all instructions when boarding, never jumping into line before his time. He assists his beleaguered parents by carrying his own bags. While maneuvering the slim aisle of an aircraft, a young gentleman is aware of other passengers trying to maneuver their carry-on bags overhead or under their seats. He does not, though he is smaller, squeeze past them but waits, and if he is of sufficient size, he offers to help. Once at his row he gathers and stows those things he has brought to occupy himself on

TRAVELING MANNERS

the flight and quickly takes his seat to allow other passengers to pass. If another passenger comes along to occupy the vacant window seat in his row, a young gentleman gets up to let that person squeeze in.

While some airlines have recently widened the seat cushion and added more knee room, the fact remains that every passenger, no matter his size, is allotted about two square feet of space. A young gentleman does not sprawl in his seat but keeps his knees no more than a couple of inches apart. Most airline seats can be moved to a reclining position. It is considerate to ask the person behind you if they mind you reclining your seat. As there is little difference in the two positions (reclined and upright), a young gentleman shouldn't need to recline the seat anyway. A young gentleman never kicks the back of the seat in front of him, pulls on it to hoist himself up, or takes more than one armrest.

A young gentleman responds politely when spoken to by a fellow passenger, but by opening a book or putting on headphones, he can signal that he would prefer not to carry on a lengthy conversation about his grades and extracurricular activities. A young man does not call the harried flight attendant for frivolous matters, nor does he ask the flight attendant to recite the beverage menu, bring him more ice, or exchange his turkey sandwich for ham. He does not ask a fellow passenger if he is going to eat his cookie. A young gentleman puts on headphones if he is using anything with volume, which he keeps low enough that his fellow passengers can't hear. He does not sing along with the music only he hears.

When the plane lands, a young gentleman resists the urge to imitate fellow passengers who do not believe rules apply to them but remains seated until the plane is secured at the gate and the seat belt sign is turned off. He retrieves his carry-ons as efficiently as possible and offers to help other passengers if he is able. At the luggage carousel, a young gentleman does not push in front of others to get his bag.

Rules of air travel generally apply to other modes of long-distance transportation, such as trains and buses.

When staying at a hotel, a young gentleman remembers that he is not the only guest. He does not treat the lobby as a gymnasium or ride up and down in the glass elevator as if it were an amusement park ride. When boarding an elevator, he waits until all disembarking passengers exit, then he moves as far to the back as possible after pushing the button for his floor. If he is already inside and closest to the control panel, he might hold the doors for others to get in safely and ask them what floor they would like. He does not punch all the buttons on an elevator or push the alarm or emergency stop button to see what will happen. He does not talk on the elevator emergency phone.

In his room he remembers that there are other guests beside, above, and below him. He does not jump on the bed; turn the television or radio up exceedingly loud; bounce a ball off the floor, ceiling, or walls; slam drawers and doors; or roughhouse with his siblings.

When riding in a taxi, a young gentleman gets in first and slides across the seat, saving less agile adults the trouble. He allows the adult to give the driver their destination, and does not make fun of the driver's accent or name posted on his license. He takes all his belongings out of the cab when they reach their destination.

When taking public transportation, a young gentleman has his fare card or exact change ready at the turnstile or door of the bus so as not to delay other riders. He takes a seat if one is available. If one is not, he finds a way to secure his position so that sudden movements do not send him flying into another rider's lap. If he has a seat on a full bus, and an elderly person or a woman with small children boards, a young gentleman gets up and offers his seat. When his stop is imminent, a young man prepares to disembark and moves through the mass without shoving, saying "Excuse me" as needed.

When going through a door, a young gentleman makes sure not to allow the door to slam on the person behind him. Instead, he holds it open for that person to catch. If he is strong enough, a young gentleman can open the door for others and let them pass through. A young gentleman does not play in revolving doors or stop them to trap a sibling or friend inside. He does

not push them around so quickly that someone might
get hurt.

You Know You Are Raising
a Gentleman If . . .

He presents a neat appearance and maintains
control of his belongings when traveling.

He does not try to sneak a pocketknife through
security or make jokes about weapons to the
security officer.

He makes correct use of the pillows and blanket
offered by the flight attendant, and does not
confuse his seat for a bed.

He does not try repeatedly to open a restroom
door that is clearly occupied in an attempt to
hurry the occupant.

He leaves the lavatory in better condition than he
found it.

He does not bring on board a plane messy foods or
ones with very strong odors.

He keeps the volume of what he is listening to on
headphones at a level only he can hear, and turns
it off during take-off or landing.

He turns off the volume on his computer and
handheld games.

Parent Pointers

Present a neat appearance and maintain control of your belongings.

Do all you can to be certain your own children are sitting with you and not with the nice elderly lady ten rows back.

Do not bury your head in a book or your laptop and tune out your son; he is your responsibility. The flight attendant is not a babysitter.

Bring along compact diversions for small boys, and allow an older boy to pack his own backpack.

Be sure to let him know what is and is not permitted in a carry-on bag, and prepare yourself and your children to go through security efficiently and not delay other passengers.

Present a good example to your children by following air industry policies and regulations, no matter how frustrated you may be by canceled flights, lost luggage, and snippy personnel.

Do not assume that a boy under the age of six can master the intricacies of an airplane bathroom by himself.

Do not succumb to horn blowing, ranting, vulgar physical gestures, or other unmistakable signs of road rage in the car.

Instruct your son to stand up and offer his seat on a crowded bus or subway.

Always open doors for the elderly and mothers pushing strollers or carrying babies.

TRY THIS AT HOME

If your son is going to be flying solo—to visit a grandparent or a noncustodial parent—you must thoroughly prepare him beforehand. Tell him what will be expected of him, and go over all the above rules of mannerly travel. Be sure he knows that while rules of talking to strangers are relaxed on an airplane, if a fellow passenger says or does anything inappropriate to him or makes him uncomfortable in any way, he should get up from his seat and privately inform a flight attendant immediately. He should never go with anyone who has not been pre-authorized by you, even if that person says you have sent them. Most airlines prohibit children twelve and under from anything but nonstop flights.

SOME GOOD ADVICE

On a flight from Dallas to Gunnison, Colorado, bad weather forced our landing in Colorado Springs instead. We sat on the runway for five hours before flying back to Dallas. The flight, like most these days, didn't provide even a boxed meal. People were famished, a condition that in addition to the stale air, the confined space, and the lengthy delay, led to extreme crankiness. One mother had packed boxes of raisins and some granola bars in a bag for her own three children, and she generously shared with two other children on board. Another passenger contributed some chewing gum to the kids, and another had Lifesavers, so they were content for a good portion of the time. In these days of delays and cancellations, never board a flight without a supply of snacks for your kids (or extra diapers if you are still using them). A flight that starts out as an hour could easily be stretched to four or five, and not only will your kids be happier if you are prepared, but also your fellow passengers will be grateful.

Chapter Eleven

WHEN NATURE CALLS: BATHROOMS, BELCHING, BOOGERS, GAS, SPITTING, AND SCRATCHING

From time to time, nature calls on all of us to attend to certain needs. Nowhere is the great divide between the genders more evident than in how each sex attends to these needs.

Generally, girls treat such needs privately and even consider them a little bit embarrassing, while boys regard them as a reason for public celebration. A young girl may very well be capable of belching the alphabet, but rarely do we witness one showing off that particular talent in public. Think of the mayhem that would ensue at Junior Miss Pageants if that were the case.

On the other hand, a boy who has mastered this stupid human trick is much admired by other boys. I know this because my son is one of those boys, something I discovered while driving him and two of his friends to a baseball game (where they could observe two additional and uniquely masculine skills: spitting and scratching). Belching the alphabet is not my son's only gift; he can also make loud noises under his arm and under his knee.

There is no argument that children's television and movies have become more vulgar, with a disturbing inclination toward bathroom humor. Once they reach adolescence, boys can avail themselves of a questionable entertainment genre entirely devoted to gross-out humor.

Even without exposure to wide-screen glorification of what is better carried out behind closed doors—or at least with some discretion—young boys will find all "bathroom" words infinitely amusing and irrationally hilarious. It's annoying but not alarming. Belching and passing gas are also natural, and a young boy should never be shamed for the act itself.

If a young gentleman has mastered the art of belching the alphabet, there is no way he is not going to show off that achievement to his friends. He does not, however, perform the stunt in a classroom, his parent's office, a place of worship, a restaurant, during a party, for his grandmother's bridge club, or anywhere else people may be offended. In other words, belching the alphabet should be an exclusive and command performance open only to a select few, in very private locations.

If a young man accidentally belches or passes gas in public or in a small group, the mild offense can be resolved by simply saying, "Excuse me." No elaboration is necessary. If someone else passes gas or belches, a young gentleman does not laugh uproariously, point fingers, one-up the offender, or make crude remarks. If a young gentleman knows he is going to belch, he keeps his lips closed to prevent a cacophonous expulsion, and if he feels the dire need to pass gas, a young gentleman can excuse himself to a bathroom or an area far enough away from his company to spare them discomfort.

There is no doubt that boys have more fun learning to pee in the toilet than girls—every time is like target practice. Still, young men should keep something in mind that someone has to clean the toilet, and since it typically is not him, the courteous thing to do is keep his urine where it belongs—in the toilet bowl. When using a bathroom that is not equipped with a urinal, a boy puts the seat up before urinating and back down when he is finished. If he still gets the seat wet, he should wipe it off with a piece of toilet paper.

When a young gentleman uses a public restroom, he closes the door to the stall, flushes after use, and then washes his hands. He uses a towel rather than the seat of his pants for drying and places the towel back where he found it or puts discarded paper towels in the trash (the general vicinity of the trash can does not count).

For completely inexplicable reasons, many very young boys get into the habit of not only picking their noses but also tasting the contents. This should be discouraged early and often. Everyone at one time or another feels the need to remove something from his nose. Even in private it is a good idea for a young man to get into the habit of executing this with discretion or using a tissue to explore the inner reaches.

Scratching and spitting are two habits of questionable taste that are also nearly always the exclusive domain of the male gender. Both seem to have something to do with professional athletes, particularly baseball players. They not only engage in these practices regularly but also often on television and the stadium JumboTron, with little regard for modesty or decorum. One might theorize that the reason for scratching has to do with the protective support equipment athletes must wear. Spitting is obviously the only effective method for getting rid of noxious chewing tobacco juice or the hulls of sunflower seeds. Even so these on-field habits nearly always travel off-field as well. Young boys naturally emulate professional athletes, and even the ones who are years away from using protective gear or chewing tobacco will imitate their heroes. It is certainly a parent's responsibility in teaching good manners to ask for more discretion when attending to itches and to insist on no unnecessary or exhibition spitting in public.

YOU KNOW YOU ARE RAISING A GENTLEMAN IF . . .

He squelches his belches in public and leaves the room if he feels the need to pass gas. He should say, "Excuse me," if he should unexpectedly or unavoidably do either in the company of others.

He employs accurate aim toward toilet bowls. If an accident occurs, he wipes the seat but does not put paper towels in the toilet.

He puts the seat down after use.

He cleans out the sink after use.

He uses a small amount of air freshener, if one is available, when his visit to the bathroom results in a lingering odor.

He does not glorify his own personal habits or call attention to those of others.

He uses a tissue or handkerchief with discretion to clear his nose of annoying obstructions.

He does not treat spitting as a competitive sport but as a means to rid himself of excess nasal drip, and then only with certainty as to the targeted receptacle.

He does not scratch his groin in view of others, but instead he turns his back if he has an itch to tend to.

Parent Pointers

Employ the same good personal habits you seek from your son.

Do not engage in immature competitions with your son, as they encourage crude behavior.

Be aware of the vulgar nature of some children's programming and make informed decisions about what type of humor to which you are exposing your child.

Do not laugh at belching and farting.

Do not laugh at, nor appear too horrified by, your son's ability to belch "Happy Birthday," but impress upon him the rudeness of doing it in public.

TRY THIS AT HOME

Leaving the room, or at least the dinner table, is what a young man should do if he knows he needs to pass gas. If he is in his classroom, church, a restaurant, or an airplane, he can excuse himself to go to the bathroom. But what if he is in a car? It would be impractical and silly to pull over every time he needs to pass gas. Instead, in our car, my children issue a warning. When one of them says, "Safety," we all roll down our windows.

SOME GOOD ADVICE

One of my friends has two boys. She told me she toilet trained the first one just before he turned three during the summer at the beach. She simply allowed him to pee outside—against a tree in their yard, on a sand dune, or even into the bay from their pier. She said he enjoyed the alfresco urinating experience so much that he was soon out of diapers altogether. My friend thought this was wonderful until they went back to the city. They weren't there five minutes before her son was peeing on a tree in the middle of a busy sidewalk. It took weeks to break him of his habit of urinating au naturel. The moral of the story: potty training isn't called potty training for nothing. Unless you're lost in the woods, pee and poop go in the toilet, and that goes for grown-up boys as well.

Chapter Twelve

PRIVACY, BOUNDARIES, AND APPROPRIATE ATTIRE

A photograph that always makes me laugh whenever I run across it is of my son, his friend, and his friend's younger brother in the Jacuzzi bath at his friend's house. The two older boys were about five, the younger was around three. There are a series of shots. The photographer apparently instructed the boys to act out "See no evil, hear no evil, say no evil" with each boy taking a different part. There are bubbles everywhere, and the water is up to their chests. Until the final shot, when all three have jumped up, arms raised, in a "ta-da!" moment, grinning from ear to soapy ear, gloriously, joyfully naked as jaybirds.

The photo still makes my son smile when he sees it, remembering the fun they had. But he also made me swear not to use it in the photo collage for his senior page in the high school yearbook. His friend extracted the same promise from his mother regarding his bar mitzvah.

In my experience of parenting a girl and a boy, I can generalize that boys come to modesty later than girls. I can't recall often, if ever, having to say, "Please put some clothes on!" to my daughter. On the other hand, I can't count the number of times I walked past my son's bedroom and saw him sitting on the floor, engrossed in building a new K'NEX structure, still totally naked from the bathtub he left thirty minutes before. "Please put some clothes on!" Eventually, his need for privacy began to keep pace with the trajectory of his development.

Young boys often disguise or assimilate their curiosity and growing awareness of sexuality and changing bodies with humor. I could not say the words "nuts" or "balls," or the name "Dick," to my son and his pals without gales of laughter in response. But educating your son about his body, boundaries, sexuality, and appropriate behavior is serious. If you are unsure where, when, and how to begin, there are many books and plenty of information on the Internet. Parents can and should discuss with their pediatrician when and how to talk about sexuality with their son.

Conversations about reproduction and human sexuality are an ongoing process, and should be addressed openly, honestly, positively—and appropriate to their age. There is no reason to have the same conversation with a six-year-old that you would with a sixteen-year-old.

It can begin with teaching young men the correct word for sexual organs—penis, testicles, vagina, breasts, and rectum. Young boys generally delight in using locker room words, but they need to know it is not appropriate to use them in public, in front of adults, or in mixed company.

Before your son starts preschool, explain to him in a relaxed but firm tone what "private parts" and "inappropriate touching" mean. By nature, children are curious and exploratory. They also want to please others, particularly grown-ups they like and trust. He needs to hear from his parents—with reinforcement from the pediatrician on annual checkups—what is normal and appropriate, what is not, and how to say "no".

While a mother can and should talk to her son about sex, this is an ideal time for a father to have a talk with his son about sex, love, physicality, personal habits, respect for women, and that "no" means "no".

Children develop at different ages, but typically girls develop before boys, and girls are reaching puberty at an earlier age than ever before. Boys must know it is not appropriate to remark on girls' developing bodies, to point, stare, and giggle, or ever to touch.

A young gentleman does not exhibit his private parts to others, nor does he show off a state of arousal. A young gentleman does not touch other children—boys or girls—on their private parts or ask them to touch his. He does his own sexual exploration in the privacy of his bedroom or bathroom and does not share his discoveries with others.

Young gentlemen do not wear T-shirts or caps printed with vulgar or offensive comments. The practice of sagging—allowing pants to slip well below the waistline so that one's underwear is visible—is not allowed in most schools and is considered offensive to many. A young gentleman dresses appropriate to the setting and occasion, whether it is church, school, or the dinner table. He does not come to the table without a shirt, and he removes his cap before sitting down.

You Know You Are Raising a Gentleman If . . .

He does not defy his school's dress code, and wears clothing appropriate to the function he is attending and the place where it is held.

He checks his zipper before leaving the bathroom or his bedroom.

He does not laugh or point at a boy who has neglected to check his fly, but discreetly lets him know he has unfinished business.

He always knocks on a closed door, particularly one that leads to a bathroom or bedroom.

He does not use locker room words in
inappropriate places.

He does not leer at girls or women, or make
offensive and inappropriate remarks about their
looks or bodies.

He does not touch anyone else's private parts, or
allow anyone else to touch his.

Parent Pointers

Knock on your son's bedroom or bathroom door
before entering, unless there is a clear indication
of danger.

Respect your son's developing sense of modesty,
and don't embarrass him by sharing those
photos of him frolicking in his birthday suit to
other people.

Make every effort to educate your son about
sexuality, boundaries, and appropriate and
inappropriate touching in a timely and
unthreatening fashion.

Be open and receptive to questions your son may
have about his and others' sexuality, even if his
questions make you uncomfortable.

Do not make up answers to those questions, or
share deliberately false information. If you

are concerned about the nature of your son's questions, ask for advice from his pediatrician.

Use the appropriate words for sexual organs, reproduction, and sexual acts.

If a boy is accidentally discovered by a parent when he is engaged in sexual exploration, a parent does not make the boy feel ashamed of what he is doing.

Do not make inappropriate, leering, or derogatory remarks about other people's shapes and sizes or make assumptions or judgments about their sexuality,

TRY THIS AT HOME

If you are a single mother, and the time comes to begin "the talk," it can be awkward. My son is rather reserved and shy, and I knew he would be uncomfortable if I just dove right in. I did a little research on the Internet and found that there are books available at all reading levels, with material appropriate to that age group. I would simply leave the book on my son's bed, with a note inviting him to read it in the privacy of his own bedroom, and talk to me if he didn't understand something. It was easier for him to point to a passage or section of the book and ask me a question, then to initiate questions on his own.

Some Good Advice

Don't tell your children more than they want to know or are ready to hear. When your four-year-old asks where babies come from, he is not asking for a lesson on reproduction and details of sexual intercourse. He is asking a simple question that only requires a simple answer, such as, "Babies grow in a special place inside the mother." As he has seen pregnant women, or may be asking because his pregnant mother is looking as if she swallowed a basketball, this answer will satisfy him for the time being. Do not lie to your child by telling him the stork brings babies. As he gets older, he will become more curious. "How does the baby get in there? How does the baby get out?" Though we all believe that the birds-and-bees conversation is going to happen in some quiet, thoughtful, sharing way, the truth is that kids usually ask these questions at the most inconvenient times: from the backseat of the car, in the checkout line at the grocery store, or when you are on the phone. Answer his question in a truthful, straightforward, natural way. Don't tell him he is too young to ask such questions. But don't give him an answer he is too young to comprehend.

Chapter Thirteen

TEMPER TEMPER

According to child development experts, for children aged one to three, temper tantrums are a natural and predictable expression of a child's first surges of independence. It's how parents react to these early immature and often embarrassing expressions of frustration that may determine how their son learns to manage his anger in the future.

During one of our first annual Easter egg hunts, when the oldest children were still toddlers, a three-year-old boy looked in his basket and determined that he had not gotten as many plastic candy-filled eggs as he thought he deserved, though certainly no less than most of the other children. His reaction to this deprivation was to hurl himself onto the ground and throw an ear-splitting, wailing, bawling, screaming, crying, kicking, flailing fit—one of the worst ever witnessed by any parent on hand that day. The other children stared in wide-eyed, open-mouthed amazement as his face turned redder and redder and his wailing louder and louder. Many of the parents also stared in amazement as the child's parents kneeled beside him, desperately trying to appease him, promising that if he would just stop they would get him as many eggs and as much candy as he wanted. It took some time for the child to hear their supplications over his own shrieking, but eventually he quieted down and, still sniffling, accepted their offers of appeasement. A few feet away from the spectacle, some of us predicted trouble down the road.

Fast-forward a few years to Halloween night. Many of the same parents and children—including the now eight-year-old boy who had gone ballistic over the plastic eggs—were out trick-or-treating together. The ill-tempered child dillydallied, inspecting each piece of candy that he got. In an attempt to catch up with the group that was already a few houses ahead, his mother hurried him past some houses on the route. A screeching howl pierced the air. Was it a witch? A werewolf? An alien from outer space? No, it was the Monster Child who found his mother's decision completely unacceptable and expressed his disapproval by throwing another ear-splitting, wailing, bawling, screaming, crying, kicking, flailing fit. The child was old enough to talk and threw in some scathing insults along with a few "I hate you"s for good measure. As the mother attempted to placate him, the father walked away in disgust but not without a pointed barb of his own: "You've made him this way, now you do something with him!" A few feet away from the spectacle, some of us predicted a fortune in therapy.

What is wrong with this picture? Plenty. First, while every parent can expect a temper tantrum from their two- and three-year-old, giving in to the child is the worst possible method of quelling the storm—at least if you don't want to endure years and years of volcanic eruptions. When a boy under the age of three has a temper tantrum, a parent remains calm and walks away. If the tantrum takes place in public—as many do—the parent picks up the child and leaves the party, the store, the restaurant, the playground, or whatever location until the boy regains control. After the boy regains control, the parent can hold the child, explaining that although being two can be frustrating, "throwing a fit"—as they say in the South—will not result in the desired objective.

Productive parenting is united parenting. Disagreements about how to handle unruly behavior or anything else to do with child rearing should be discussed privately (or in a counselor's office) and not in front of the child.

A very young child should not be punished for what is truly a natural expression, but he should not be rewarded either. After the child turns three, a parent must let the son know in no uncertain terms that temper tantrums will not be tolerated and that not only will the child not get what he is ranting about, but that his uncontrollable behavior also will result in some type of retribution. Just as a parent helps a child learn to recite the alphabet, sing a song, and ride a bicycle, a parent is responsible—through word and deed—for teaching a son how to control his temper, handle his frustrations, and express his anger in a mature and socially acceptable manner.

A young gentleman, no matter how angry he is that he lost a video game, does not respond by smashing his fist onto the keyboard or throwing his DS across the room. A young gentleman, no matter how upset he is that he did not get the Nikes that he wanted, does not respond by deliberately trashing the shoes that his parents have bought him. A young gentleman, no matter how affronted he is when a classmate cuts in front of him in the cafeteria line, does not respond by pushing or poking. A young gentleman, no matter how frustrated he is for striking out, does not hurl his bat toward his teammate on deck and slam his batting helmet into the dugout.

Even grown-ups lose patience and get upset when things don't go their way or seem unfair. Every person, young and old, will sometimes engage in impetuous behavior that he or she will later have cause to regret. The measure of a mature person is how they react to challenging and difficult situations.

An apology takes just a moment, but hastens forgiveness and has a lasting effect on relationships. If a young man loses his temper and, in expressing his anger, does or says something that hurts another, he first allows himself a moment to cool down, then offers a sincere, in-person apology whenever possible. If face-to-face contact is not possible, then telephoned or written amends can be substituted. If, in his anger, his actions result in something being damaged or broken, his apology must be accompanied by an offer to make reparations.

A young man learns this because he sees his parents apologize when they lose their tempers or say angry, hurtful words. He learns this because when his parents see that their son is losing control, they intervene. He learns this because when he does lose control, his parents insist he apologize, and until he does, he will remain in his room.

You Know You Are Raising a Gentleman If . . .

He does not express anger, disappointment, or frustration by using bad language or insulting someone.

He does not express anger, disappointment, or frustration by throwing, kicking, punching, or breaking something.

If he is very angry and feels that he is losing control, he goes to his room and punches or yells into his pillow if that helps.

He apologizes as soon as possible when he loses control and it affects someone else.

He does not shout to get someone's attention.

He never uses words like "fatso," "stupid," "butthead," "idiot," "porky," or "retard" when addressing another.

He does not use racial, ethnic, or sexual slurs to express himself.

Parent Pointers

Do not respond to a temper tantrum by giving in to a child's tantrum or promising to get him a treat if he stops.

If your son is having a temper tantrum in a public place or around other people, take him to another room or outside.

Do not react to your son's bad behavior with similar bad behavior, such as hitting a child to stop him from hitting.

Do your best not to raise your voice in anger to a child, unless a child is in danger.

Do not yell at other people or question their parenting in front of their children.

Do not call other people names. Even if you think the driver who just made a left turn from the far right lane is an idiot, you are only stating the obvious if you announce it.

If you curse or use vulgarities in front of your children, don't be surprised when they begin using the same words. It sounds just as bad coming from your mouth as it does from theirs.

Do not throw golf clubs, tennis rackets, bats, books, jewelry, or anything else in anger.

If you lose your temper with your child, apologize.

Accept apologies quickly and graciously when they are made to you.

Part of forgiving is forgetting. Once someone apologizes and you accept the apology, it is over. Let it go.

TRY THIS AT HOME

When I became a mom, I made a conscious effort to stop cursing, especially around the children, but it happens. Sometimes I'm not even aware of it myself. They may overhear me on the telephone or in a conversation with a friend, and they are quick to point out my infraction. We have a "fine" jar, and every time I use a curse word, I have to deposit a quarter. Similarly, if my children tell someone to "shut up", or call someone "stupid", they are fined as well. Once a year, we use the change for a good cause, such as buying books or toys for a family shelter or domestic violence center or adopting a needy family at

Christmas. The rule is that you cannot use the money collected from your bad behavior to reward yourself.

Some Good Advice

My mother was a stay-at-home mom with five children. When the oldest—me—was nine, the youngest was born. She had a group to ride herd on and plenty of opportunities for discipline. I was often the recipient of her fierce attention, but every time she was forced to have words with me, she did it privately. I do not recall my mother ever admonishing or punishing us in public or in front of our friends. There were times, if my behavior was extreme, that she sent my friends home, so that she could send me to my room, but she did it in a very simple way: "Mary, we're glad you came to play, but Kay needs some time by herself. We'll see you tomorrow." Avoid disciplining your child in public or in front of anyone else.

Chapter Fourteen

RELIGION, POLITICS, AND SANTA CLAUS

The cardinal rule of convivial dinner parties is to avoid discussing religion or politics. That may be prudent, but it could make for a pretty dull evening. Surely mature adults can be counted upon to engage in thoughtful discourse on stimulating and controversial topics with respect and regard for opinions that differ from their own.

In reality, since otherwise mature adults are not always capable of this, we can hardly expect it of our children. Does that mean, in order to be mannerly, subjects that may spark disagreement must be avoided? Not necessarily, but boys should be taught that opinions are like noses: everybody has one, but none of them are exactly the same. Just because somebody's opinion is different doesn't make them wrong or stupid or idiotic.

In most parts of the world it is considered bad manners to ask someone what their religious affiliation is or where they attend church. In the South it is perfectly natural in the course of casual conversation between adults for a new acquaintance to inquire, "Where did you go to school? What do you do? Where do you live? Where do you go to church?" For many people in the South going to church is as much social as it is spiritual. (It's called the Bible Belt for a reason.) A young man might, out of curiosity, ask his new friend where he attends church, but he does not make a negative comment in response. A young Methodist gentleman does not tell his Catholic friend he thinks confession is weird, nor does an Evangelical Christian gentleman warn his Jewish classmate that he is going straight to hell unless he accepts Jesus as his Savior.

A young man may invite a friend to attend church or temple with him. He does not insist that his friend participate in any part of the service that is not comfortable for him. Likewise, if a young man attends church or temple with a friend of a different religious persuasion, he is respectful of the service and practices, but he is not required to participate in communion, testimony, the laying on of hands, or even singing.

In situations where a public prayer is said, a young gentleman who does not subscribe to the theology of the assembled does not make a display of his differences but shows respect by remaining quiet through the prayer. If grace is said before a meal at which he is a guest, he does not announce that his family does not say grace; he simply bows his head. If the family holds hands around the table, he participates without comment.

In recent years, political campaigns have become more contentious, accusatory, and divisive. Extensive news coverage of even the most mundane details, and endless cycles of attack ads expose children to the uglier aspects of politics. While it's often disturbing enough to make us all turn to ESPN or QVC, it can present an opportunity for parents and teachers to offer children lessons in fairness, civic responsibility, and respect for people of differing opinions and stances.

Many schools participate in a program called Kids Vote, which allows children to register their choice of candidates as well as wear candidate paraphernalia in the weeks leading up to the actual election. A young gentleman does not mock another child's choice or political affiliation or make disparaging comments about his or her candidate. He does not accuse the other candidate of cheating in order to win, nor does he gloat if his candidate wins.

If a boy holds strong beliefs about a subject— from the designated hitter rule to global warming or capital punishment—he does not try to impose his beliefs on others, nor make fun of those whose beliefs differ from his own. He can express his thoughts on a controversial topic if he can do so in a non-confrontational and non-contentious manner.

On the subject of Santa Claus, the Tooth Fairy, and the Easter Bunny: when a young gentleman discovers or is told the truth about these childhood fantasies, he should not share this with other children who may still be captivated by their magic. Soon after his seventh Christmas, my son came to me and asked, with a fair degree of trepidation, if Santa Claus was real. I responded in the time-honored parental response to tough questions: "What do you think?" He, rather wistfully and somewhat hopeful of a positive response, said, "I don't think he is." It was all I could do not to burst into tears, but as he was on the verge himself, I very gently replied, "Do you mean that you don't believe there is a jolly fat man who lives on the North Pole with Mrs. Claus and hundreds of little elf helpers who make millions of toys all year long, then pack them into a little sleigh that is pulled by eight tiny reindeer to deliver all those presents in a single night to good boys and girls all over the world?" Even he had to laugh at the image, which helped diffuse the disappointment. I told him that believing in Santa Claus was a wonderful, magical thing that children and their parents love to celebrate for as long as possible. I also asked him to remember the meaning of Christmas as we personally observe it as members of the Episcopal Church.

He nodded his head solemnly and then asked the Big Question: "Does this mean I won't get any presents anymore?" After I assured him that he would still get presents under the tree and a stocking by the fireplace as long as he wanted, his next concern was keeping it a secret from his sister, who happens to be nearly two years older than him, and had known for almost that long the truth about Santa. I pointed out to him how generous it had been of her to help me keep that fantasy alive for him until he discovered the truth himself, and that he was now charged with that same responsibility when it came to children younger than him. He walked away from the conversation feeling very happy. I closed my office door and shed a few tears for one more piece of his childhood gone forever.

You Know You Are Raising a Gentleman If . . .

He does not make fun of, scoff, or pass judgment on another person's religious beliefs or practices.

He is respectful when attending a religious service with a friend of a different theology.

He bows his head and is respectful of a blessing before a meal, wherever and whenever it is said.

He does not make ugly comments or accusations about another person's candidate of choice. He does not make fun of another person's political affiliation.

He does not impose his spiritual or political beliefs on others.

Parent Pointers

Do not make comments or pass judgment in front of your children about another's spiritual or political beliefs.

Do not make a guest in your home or place of worship engage in practices that are uncomfortable for him or her.

Do not say horrid or hateful things about politicians or community leaders.

Do not call elected officials names. Whether you voted for the president of the United States or not, he or she is still the president of the country. The office deserves our respect.

Try This at Home

If your son comes home from school and tells you an Indian child has joined his classroom, or he is invited to dine with a Korean family, do some research with him on the unfamiliar country and culture. At the end of our street is the Islamic Center, a place of worship and community for Muslims in our city. Once a quarter, they hold an open house and bake sale, and we always attend. It gives us the opportunity to meet our neighbors, and them an opportunity to teach us about their faith and worship services. We love trying the foods the women of the Center prepare, and it gives my kids a chance to play with children of the Muslim faith. When unfamiliar cultures are personalized, they cease to be strange or threatening, and your children will see that people of the world are more alike than different.

SOME GOOD ADVICE

Voting is more than a right; it's a responsibility of every American. I vote in every election, from school board to presidential, and since my children have been babies, I have taken them to the polls with me, pulling their strollers into the voting booth. As soon as they were old enough to reach, I let them push the buttons and pull the lever. Now that they are reading, we look over the sample ballot in the newspaper before election day, and I wait until they are home from school so they can come with me. They look forward to it and even more to the day when they can vote themselves. As we saw in the contested 2000 election, every vote really does count.

Chapter Fifteen

TELEPHONE MANNERS

L ook in any playroom, preschool, or day care center and you will probably find toy phones and cell phones. Children love to imitate their parents by playing telephone, making a game of punching buttons, and babbling away in an imaginary conversation. But in every child's life there comes a time when he or she must be taught the difference between a toy telephone and the real deal. The telephone may be the best and most efficient way to reach out and touch someone, but with such easy access to people's homes, it can also be irritatingly intrusive. Cell phones are so accessible and widespread as to seem ubiquitous and nearly inescapable.

Many households have eliminated their landline phones altogether, relying solely on their mobile devices. Generally though, older people who have a hard time letting go of their comfort zones, and homes with school-age children who want a common family phone hold on to their landlines.

With the exception of knowing how, when, and why to dial 911, a child should not be permitted to answer the phone or place calls until he knows how to do it properly. It is also important that your child is articulate enough that he can be understood by the caller or callee and can accurately take a message in the event the parent is unavailable. Fortunately, instructions for proper use of the telephone are fairly simple and can be rehearsed on a toy telephone.

A young gentleman answers the telephone in his own home in one of the following ways: "Hello," "Hello, Carter residence, Martin speaking," or "Carter residence, this is Martin." The caller may say something like, "Hello, Martin, this is Mrs. West. May I speak with your mother, please?" Depending on the circumstances, Martin might say, "I'm sorry, she isn't available right now. May I take a message?" or "Just a moment, please." A young gentleman would then—this is very important—either put the receiver down and find his mother or cover the receiver with his hand and call his mother to the phone. He does not yell "Mom!" into the telephone.

If his parents are not at home, he does not reveal the absence of an adult. Instead, he says, "She is not able to come to the phone," and offers to take a message. Phones should have a pad of paper and writing implement nearby. A young gentleman takes the caller's name and a number where the caller can be reached. He writes the information legibly on the pad.

When a young gentleman places a call from his home phone, he speaks clearly and loudly enough to be heard: "Hello, this is Marshall. May I speak to Malcolm, please?" If Malcolm is not available or not at home, a young gentleman then says, "Would you please ask him to call Marshall? My number is 234-5678. Thank you."

A young man is prepared to leave a message with a voice mail system, as most phones are equipped with them. When a phone is answered by machine or voice mail, a young man speaks clearly, audibly, and slowly. Make the message short. "Hello, this is Marshall. Please have Malcolm call me at 234-5678. Thank you."

Answering systems are designed to take messages. Overly cute but barely decipherable outgoing messages that cause people to hang up defeat the purpose of the system. Unless your child can articulate the greeting on your answering machine, leave it to an adult or a computer. If your child can clearly say something like, "This is 798-1700, please leave a message," without giggling, he is ready to record the outgoing announcement, though that doesn't mean he should.

A young gentleman does not monopolize the home's only telephone line; time limits can be set on children's phone calls. If a home phone is equipped with call waiting, a child knows how to operate it. If he is on the phone when another call beeps in, he defers to the incoming call, lest it be his parent's boss calling to tell him the presentation deadline has been moved up. When another call beeps into his, he says, "Please hold on a moment." He takes the next call and if it is for one of his parents, he asks the incoming caller to hold for a moment, goes back to the first call, and asks if he might call back.

A young gentleman does not place phone calls during inconvenient times, such as the dinner hour, roughly 5:30–7:00 p.m. He does not call a home before 8:00 a.m. or after 8:00 p.m. on weekdays, nor before 10:00 a.m. or after 9:00 p.m. on weekends.

If a young gentleman inadvertently dials a wrong number, he does not hang up when recognizing that fact, but instead says, "I'm sorry, I must have dialed a wrong number." If he is not sure, a young man says, "Is this 234-5678?" He does not ask the person answering the phone what number he has called, and if the reverse occurs, he does not give out his telephone number to someone he doesn't know.

A young gentleman is aware that cell phones are expensive and that no matter how cute they are, they are not toys. Unless he has been given permission to do so, a young gentleman does not place calls on his parents' cell phone. He does not give his parents' cell phone numbers to his buddies. If he is asked to make or take a call on a cell phone, he knows how to disconnect calls. Many parents are giving their children cell phones at a fairly young age, particularly if work or travel separates them from their children for long periods of time. The ground rules for the use of cell phones should be preset and firm. In the first stages of cell phone ownership, you might set a rule that he is only allowed to call his parents on the cell phone, not every buddy in his sixth-grade class. Let him know that you can and will monitor incoming and outgoing calls.

Children with cell phones must know and practice proper etiquette. A young gentleman turns the volume off in movie theaters, school, and church, and does not talk or text in any of those places, or at the table. He shouldn't use the cell phone for talking or texting when his full attention is required for his safety, such as on a bicycle. Misuse of the instruments should result in their confiscation.

You Know You Are Raising a Gentleman If . . .

He speaks clearly and audibly on the telephone and knows how to take and leave a message.

He does not yell "Mom!" directly into the receiver when the caller has asked for his mother, nor does he chomp gum or food while on the phone.

He knows to turn the volume down or the cell phone off in movie theaters, performance halls, at church, or in school.

He does not talk loudly on his cell phone in common areas so that everyone is privy to his private conversation.

He does not text incessantly when he is in the presence of actual people.

He does not call too early in the morning or too late at night.

He does not hog the family telephone.

He does not chew gum or food or cough into a telephone.

He does not disregard calls coming in on a shared line while he is on another call, nor ignore the original caller.

He returns the portable phone to its receiver.

He does not answer the phone in someone else's house.

He does not place a call from someone else's house without their permission.

He does not place prank or obscene calls; besides being rude, it is also illegal.

Parent Pointers

Teach your son how, when, and why to use 911. Give him some examples of the differences between a real emergency (the house across the street is on fire) and a problem (the cat is up the tree and can't get down).

Make sure your son knows his home phone number and when it is appropriate to share it.

Teach your son how to answer and place calls properly. Until he has mastered the task, do not allow him to use the phone except in an emergency.

Teach your son how to use telephone amenities such as call-waiting and voice mail.

Do not chew gum or food while on the phone.

Do not be rude to telephone solicitors. If you don't want to be bothered, cut them off promptly and politely and ask to have your name removed from their calling list.

Turn your cell phone to vibrate or off in confined public places like restaurants, waiting rooms, and libraries. If you must make or take a call, excuse yourself and converse privately.

Do not drive and talk on the cell phone simultaneously. It is dangerous and illegal in many states.

Do not drive and text. It almost certainly is illegal and can have tragic consequences.

Do not ask your son to lie on your behalf by telling a caller you are not available when you simply do not want to take the call.

Try This at Home

Help your son understand that there is no such thing as "free" when it comes to cell phone service. If you provide your son with his own cell phone, you will certainly want to get on a family plan right away to allow for the increased number of minutes and texts that will accrue as a result of another user. Parents should check monthly bills thoroughly for extra fees, and go over itemized charges with your son until he gets it. New users often sign up for services delivered over their cell phones without realizing they involve a fee. Be sure they know that not even directory assistance is free.

Some Good Advice

On the rare moments when a girl isn't using her cell phone, she can carry it in her purse. Boys have no recourse other than their pockets, which results in torn pockets, unintended calls, and dropped or lost phones. Nothing can be done about the pockets, but I found the insurance I added to my son's phone was a wise investment and paid itself back after he dropped his first phone in the creek he and his friends were exploring, and his second fell out of his back pocket while he was riding the Ferris wheel at the state fair.

Chapter Sixteen

COMPUTERS, THE INTERNET, AND SOCIAL MEDIA

Among the four phones in our home is a black antique rotary phone I kept in the family room, on top of a side table next to the sofa. It was more for the effect than function, as we typically used either the wall phone in the kitchen, or one of the two portable phones. One evening, watching the Little League World Series in the family room, my son asked if he could call his Little League teammate to come over and watch with us. When I said yes, he began to get up from the sofa to go get a phone, and I casually said, "Just use that one," pointing to the rotary. The complete puzzlement on his face was priceless, as he lifted the heavy receiver and pondered the round thing with the numbers. He looked at me in some dismay, and said, "What do I do?"

That's pretty much the same reaction I had the first time I sat down in front of a computer. "What do I do?" Our children, on the other hand, seem to have been born with a computer chip already implanted in their brains. That doesn't mean they don't need a user manual and that there isn't an occasional malfunction.

Computer use begins well before preschool, and even pre-readers develop skills that put their parents, and certainly their grandparents, to shame. Having and knowing how to operate a computer or mobile operating system opens the door to a vast universe of information and communication, but can also be the window to a world of trouble.

Because I work at home and my computer is a crucial tool to my livelihood, my desktop computer has always been off-limits to my children. The family computer—one I traded up from—is the one they use, on a table in a common room where I can keep an eye on them.

There are many options in parental control software, easily researched online, with various levels of monitoring. I strongly recommended installing them on the computer your son will be using. Schools use control software as well to prevent students from going to inappropriate or unsafe sites. As your son gets older and proves to be a responsible user, his access can be expanded.

But even the most stringent control systems can be circumvented, and supervision isn't necessarily as strict in other homes as it is in your own. Parental control software does not absolve parents of the task of explaining responsible use of computers, the Internet, and social media to their children. In today's world, it is as important as "the talk" about the birds and the bees, which some boys attempt to find on the Internet, though often what they do find is not exactly the "sex education" you had in mind. Online pornography today is extreme, graphic, crude, intensely vulgar, often violent, and has nothing to do with love, affection, or respect—qualities parents hope their sons will find in their future relationships.

Often boys stumble on these sites unknowingly and can be very confused and even frightened by what they see. Be sure to check the history on the family computer search engine on a regular basis to see where you son has been. Monitoring the history on the family computer isn't just to keep an eye out for pornography, but for any site you feel is too old for your son, inappropriate, or possibly dangerous.

Not as crucial to their safety, but important to know, is the etiquette of computers and social media. Young gentlemen don't monopolize the family computer, no matter how compelling the game of Club Penguin is. He doesn't use the keyboard after eating a piece of fried chicken without washing his hands first. Young gentlemen don't place a beverage without a lid beside the keyboard. Young gentlemen know that electronics represent a sizable investment and are careful when using them. Young gentlemen don't use someone else's computer or laptop without permission.

When children start school and their circle of friends widens, they will want to communicate with them outside of school. Before computers, that was done on the family telephone. Now there are many options available, and it is up to parents which of those their son can access and when is the right age.

Increasingly, schools and teachers are using e-mail to communicate homework assignments, test scores, grades, schedule changes, and general announcements. The grade level at which students are included in that communication is up to the particular school your son attends, but typically, public schools will lag behind private schools in the use of technology to communicate with their student bodies.

If he is not assigned an address through his school, assist your son in setting up his first e-mail account, even if he can run circles around you when it comes to tech savvy. Make sure the address is appropriate and does not unintentionally give out too much information. There is extensive assistance available online to guide parents in assuring their son's online safety and not compromise his personal information or that of your family. Identity theft is common and is a nightmare to resolve.

Facebook was originally intended as a networking and social site for college students, and in order to set up a page, members had to have an authentic college e-mail address. That is no longer true, and everyone from your twelve-year-old babysitter to your eighty-two-year-old grandmother has a Facebook page.

Prior to getting his own Facebook page, your son might exchange messages with his friends via text applications on their iPods or Google's Buzz networking and messaging tool. There are also social network sites that have been created to provide communication exclusively between family members and family friends that might be a safe entry point for young children to social network, but as with anything, parents should thoroughly research the site.

For my kids, seventh grade marked the entry point to becoming a Facebook member and having their own e-mail accounts. Be certain your son understands that you will be monitoring his buddy lists, address book, and "friends" on Facebook. Make sure he uses the highest level of privacy setting and allows communication only with friends on his own list.

Be extremely clear in explaining to your son that saying offensive, mean, or untrue things, and sending or posting inappropriate photos is wrong. What takes only a few seconds to do, can't be taken back. A good rule for him to keep in mind is that he should not say anything online that he would not say to someone's face, and should not send a photo that he would have to hide from his parents or be ashamed if they saw it.

No doubt, as I type these words, the next big thing is being developed and will replace all the previous next big things. But the central message remains the same. It is crucial that you stay aware, informed, educated, and engaged enough to keep your son safe—from others and from his own immature judgment. That does not mean reading every message he receives, just as you wouldn't open every piece of mail addressed to him. It does mean knowing the password to his accounts and requiring him to accept you as a "friend," if only until you are confident that he understands the dangers that can lurk in shadows of the big world online.

You Know You Are Raising a Gentleman If . . .

He stops what he is doing on the computer when his mother calls him for dinner or his father asks him to take the dog out.

He does not try to circumvent the restrictions his parents place on his computer usage.

He does not say things online that he would not say to someone's face.

He does not send or post unflattering photos of others or send inappropriate photos of himself to anyone for any reason.

He does not go to sites marked "For Adults Only" or intended for users eighteen and over.

He does not go to unprotected chat rooms.

He does not accept friend requests from people he doesn't know.

He does not divulge personal information about himself or his family over the Internet or social networks.

Parent Pointers

Keep the family computer in a common room, where you can monitor when and how your son uses it.

Insist your son give you his password for any computer and social network accounts he has as a condition for being allowed to have them.

Do not read his mail or listen to his voice mail messages. Monitoring his use of the computer and social networks is a wise precaution for his safety; electronic eavesdropping and policing is invasive and counterproductive.

Detailed call lists for each cell phone line you are responsible for are available online. Check your son's list and know which numbers are in his network of friends. If anything raises a red flag, ask him about it. Don't jump to conclusions.

Do not text, check your e-mails, take or make calls while your children are talking to you, or when you are in the stands at their game or the audience of their play. Your children should not feel they are competing for your attention with your mobile device.

Try This at Home

Social networking can seem very antisocial if each member of the family is doing something separately—mom is on her Facebook page, Dad is on his laptop sending e-mails, and your son is on the family computer playing Animal Jam. Board games may not be your family thing, but why not sit down together and play a game you all like, search for places you might want to go on vacation, or take a trip around the world via Google Earth? Alternatively, set aside one night or one day in the week that the entire family unplugs. You might be surprised to find how connective disconnecting can be.

Some Good Advice

There is much information available online about keeping children safe on the Internet, particularly when they are first starting out. Some of those sites offer templates for a list of rules to go over with your kids, much like the list of house rules many families display on their refrigerator or a bulletin board in the kitchen. Download one of those lists, make adjustments to your individual family and son, then print out two copies, read it together, and then each of you sign both copies. Post one copy over the family computer and make sure he understands the consequences of breaking the "contract."

Chapter Seventeen

STARING AND DIFFERENCES

W hen my children were still toddlers, we moved into a house on a street in what is known as a "transitional neighborhood," one with lots of older homes in various states of either disrepair or renovation, and extremely diverse racially, ethnically, and socioeconomically.

An elderly friend who had spent all his life in the same small, close-knit rural community brought his truck to town for me to use the day of the move. Friends and I spent much of the day driving from my old house back to the new house, carrying furniture and boxes in and out of the house, saying hello to new neighbors as they passed by on the sidewalk or came over to introduce themselves. He sat on the porch all day, taking it all in. As dusk settled over my new street and I began to unpack boxes, my elderly friend turned to me and asked with complete innocence,

"Are you the only white people on the block?" I hid my amusement and replied, "Well, the gay couple who live in the yellow house, and the lesbian couple who live in the blue house are white. The family who lives in the brick house next door to the Islamic mosque on the corner is mixed—black and white. Other than that, I guess we are." He didn't say another word about it.

Parents—black, brown, white, yellow, or green—don't do their children any favors by surrounding them only with people who look and think and act like them. Sooner or later—unless you are like my small-town friend—they will go out into the world, and it would help them immeasurably to have had meaningful interaction with different types of people.

Parents of every race and creed teach their children—by thought, word, and deed—that while skin color, religion, ethnic background, and sexual preference contribute to who a person is, they are not everything a person is. Making generalizations and perpetuating stereotypes about people of other races or backgrounds is wrong and ignorant. Parents also, by example, show children that bigoted remarks, slurs, and jokes will not be tolerated in their presence. By simply saying, "We do not find those types of jokes amusing" or "We are offended by that way of speaking," your child will understand the importance you place on respecting and valuing all other people and hopefully follow your example. If the person making those jokes or remarks gets insulted, or persists, just walk away; do not get into an argument.

Aside from skin color and ethnic background, children will also come across people who are different from them because of physical or mental handicaps or disfigurement due to disease or accidents. This becomes far more common in the aftermath of a war, as we now see in the United States following two simultaneous wars. A small boy can be forgiven for staring and asking awkward questions that, coming from someone older, would be extremely rude: "Mommy, why can't that boy talk?" "Daddy, what is on that lady's face?" "Why does that man only have one arm?"

A parent should first tell his or her son that he must not stare, or worse, point at people different from him, but that he may quietly ask his parent a question about an obviously developmentally handicapped child or someone with a horrid facial scar or without an arm. If you don't know the specifics, an acceptable response would be that perhaps the lady suffered a terrible burn, or that the man lost his arm in an accident, and that sometimes things happen to babies even before they are born so not everyone turns out the same as everyone else. The parent also points out that handicapped people have to work harder than people who are not handicapped to do things we take for granted—like getting through doors, going up steps, tying shoes, and buttoning a shirt. A young gentleman treats handicapped children he may know as naturally as possible. A young gentleman can assist as long as he offers first and doesn't just barge in.

If he meets someone who is deaf, a young gentleman gets his attention by lightly touching his arm or shoulder. A young man does not shout at a deaf person but speaks audibly, distinctly, and does not rush his words. Many people in the deaf community have been taught to read lips, so a young gentleman should be certain his mouth is clearly visible.

If a young gentleman meets someone who is blind, there is no need to shout or help them get dressed, feed themselves, or move about. A young gentleman makes his entrance or departure known to a blind person. If a blind person has a guide dog, a young gentleman does not pet a Seeing Eye dog without permission, throw a ball, ask him to do tricks, or try to feed him a snack. The dog is his master's eyes, and to take him away from his job would be a disservice to both and could even be harmful.

A young gentleman does not ask a person in a wheelchair if he may drive it or take a ride. When speaking to a person in a wheelchair, a young gentleman makes every effort to have that conversation at eye level so that the person in the wheelchair does not get a crick in his neck. He does not try to assist the person in the wheelchair unless he is asked.

The mentally challenged can be frightening to children, so parents should make every effort to explain the condition to their child and assure him there is nothing to fear. A young gentleman treats a mentally challenged person with compassion and respect.

You Know You Are Raising
a Gentleman If . . .

He does not judge a book by its cover or a person by the color of his or her skin, his or her religion, his or her clothing, house, car, or lifestyle.

He does not ask, "Are you rich?" or "Are you poor?"

He does not engage in name-calling or disparaging jokes.

He does not stare or point at people with handicaps, disabilities, or physical defects.

He does not shout at physically disabled or mentally challenged people in an effort to be understood.

He does not act as if a handicap makes a person invisible.

He shows kindness and respect for the handicapped and the challenged.

Parent Pointers

Never make racial or ethnic slurs, even to repeat a story or quote someone else.

Be aware of the use of words or phrases that may be common but are nonetheless offensive: to "Jew someone down," to "Welsh on a bet," to "Gyp someone," or to call them an "Indian giver." Do not repeat racist, sexist, or ethnic jokes, or tolerate them in your presence.

Do not point or stare at the handicapped.

Answer as simply and clearly as possible your son's questions about people different from him.

Try This at Home

My cousin Billy was blind from birth. Once when we were visiting his family, Billy, who was about seven at the time, asked his mother for a glass of milk and she told him to get it himself. He got a glass from the cabinet, took the milk from the refrigerator, put the glass on the table, and put a finger inside the glass so he could measure how much he was pouring. Even so, the carton was full and he spilled a small amount on the table, something I, a fully sighted ten-year-old, did on a regular basis. His mother looked over and said, "For crying out loud, Billy, can't you see what you're doing?" There was dead silence for a moment and then we all laughed. Being around Billy growing up taught us not to treat him differently and that he had gifts beyond 20/20 vision. He grew up to get a PhD, and traveled the world playing music in clubs and coffeehouses.

If you have a friend or acquaintance who is handicapped in some way, that person may not mind talking to your son about his or her handicap or disability and letting your son know what life is like from their point of view. Answering your son's questions in an honest and forthright way would be a generous gift, and one that I don't imagine many would be reluctant to offer.

Some Good Advice

I have a brother-in-law who is paraplegic, and he has one of those magic wheelchairs that is quite a large contraption and needs plenty of room. We went to the grocery store one day in his specially equipped van, but every handicapped parking space was taken and remained taken for a good fifteen minutes as I circled the lot. A young woman with a small child finally came to fetch her car out of the handicapped spaced as we idled nearby. She looked at us a little sheepishly and said, "I'm sorry. I was just going in for a minute." Never, ever park in a handicapped parking space if you don't need one for a genuine handicap. Being in a hurry and toting small children is not a handicap. Being confined to a wheelchair is. Be thankful that you don't need the wheelchair and don't steal it from someone who does.

Chapter Eighteen

PREACHERS AND TEACHERS; CHURCH AND SCHOOL

I n some Christian denominations, the first experience a child might have with formal church is his baptism, a sacred moment for family and friends. The precious baby boy dons something fancy, often an heirloom baptismal gown. Proudly the parents and godparents approach the baptismal font and hand their child to the minister. The entire congregation looks on expectantly. If he is typical of most babies, the moment the holy water is poured over his head, he will burst into a startled and piercing wail, followed by angry and vigorous crying. Everyone smiles indulgently and says, "Isn't that darling?"

And it is darling, but not for long. After the baptism, the sound of a squalling infant or rambunctious toddler usually strikes a note of discord in the solemn sanctity of most services. Some churches deal with this issue by providing crying rooms in the back of the church where the parent on duty can retreat with the noisy babe in arms and remain included in the service, yet isolated from the other members of the congregation. Other churches and synagogues provide child care in another part of the building during the service, and parents are urged to take advantage of this until the maximum age limit or until such time when they feel their son is able to remain still and quiet for the hour or so required of him.

A young boy who has been entrusted to do so follows the common guidelines of courtesy while he is in church or temple. If he is not old enough to read and follow along with the order of service, a young boy brings along something unobtrusive to keep himself busy, the key word being unobtrusive. At a recent Easter service—which along with Christmas services lures folks who may not be familiar with church etiquette—my son and I were fascinated by a boy of about four who had brought along a portable Playskool garage complete with a half-dozen small vehicles. He set it up on the floor at the end of his pew and spread out nearly twelve inches into the aisle. There, sprawled in the aisle, he ran his cars in and out of service bays, filled up at the miniature pumps, and even went so far as to make a siren noise for the police car in hot pursuit of a little red Corvette. Everyone within sight and sound of the child was thankful when an alert usher hurried over to put the garage out of service. The boy began crying, and the mother, already proven to lack sound judgment and good manners, glared at the usher as if to say, "Now look what you've done!"

This is an extreme example of inappropriate play toys for a church but one that bears repeating, if just for its audacity. A pre-reader can bring a sticker book, a coloring book, or a sketchbook and some markers. He is not expected to do anything other than remain occupied and quiet for the duration. A young man does not lie down on a pew—I once accidentally sat squarely on my son's head when he had done so—or on the floor under the pew. He may write on the bulletin but must not remove all the printed material from the back of the pews to use as a coloring book or to make into paper airplanes.

When he is old enough, a young gentleman is encouraged to engage in those parts of the service that call for a congregation's participation. He does so with some semblance of attentiveness and solemnity without fidgeting or slouching. If the service takes an exceptionally long time, a young gentleman may turn to a book or sketchbook brought along for that purpose.

A young gentleman treats his clergyperson or religion teacher with respect, using the proper title: Reverend Stevenson, Father Francis, Rabbi Kantor. If your clergyperson's habit is to stand in the back of the church following the service to greet his or her parishioners, a young gentleman stops briefly with his parents and says hello, shaking hands if the clergyperson initiates the exchange.

Long before they start kindergarten, many children have accumulated years of experience in day care, mother's day out, or preschool, and are somewhat prepared for the rules and regulations of educational institutions.

A young gentleman knows that the classroom is the teacher's domain, and unless he is asked to do something that goes against his religion or customs of his people, he follows the laws of the land. Though I understand that certain progressive schools are allowing students to call teachers by their first names, this is very unusual and, in my view, ill advised. In most cases a young gentleman precedes his teacher's surname with Mr., Mrs., Miss, or Ms. A young gentleman treats every member of the administration and staff—from the principal to the cafeteria workers—with the utmost respect.

A young gentleman does nothing to disturb the teacher's study plan or other members of his class. He completes his assignments from the evening before and is prepared every morning with the necessary school supplies. He sits in his own seat and does not invade the physical space of his classmates or take any of their supplies without permission. He does not chatter while the teacher is teaching or while others are working. He never copies from a classmate's paper.

In the cafeteria he remembers his table manners and does not take food from another child or make unkind remarks about another child's food or eating habits. He never throws food, and he cleans up after himself in the instructed fashion.

On the playground a young gentleman waits his turn for swings and hanging bars and follows rules of play in whatever game is being played. He stops his play when recess is over and does not cause unnecessary aggravation for the playground supervisor by lagging behind.

You Know You Are Raising a Gentleman If . . .

He does not chew gum loudly in church or the classroom.

He does not talk out of turn at school.

He does not make fun of a classmate's answer to a teacher's question or a classmate's inability to answer a question.

He does not make fun of a classmate's grades on a test or report card.

When he needs to go to the restroom during church or temple, he does not disturb others on his route or dillydally on the way back.

He does not wear a hat or cap in church, but wears a yarmulke into a synagogue, even if he is not of the Jewish faith.

He addresses clergy and school staff by the appropriate titles.

He keeps his own place standing in line, never cutting in, and not pushing those ahead of him or holding up those behind.

Parent Pointers

Do not impose unruly children on fellow congregants.

Supply small boys with something to occupy them during the service. Do not supply your child with toys and diversions that will disturb others.

Dress appropriately for church. Chic hats for women are fine; hats for men—other than yarmulkes—are not.

Do not whisper, chitchat, or giggle with your spouse, friends, or children during the service.

Pay attention to the service, including the sermon, and do not use the time as an opportunity to balance your checkbook, check your e-mails, or text. Encourage your son to participate in the service when he is old enough.

Address the clergy with their proper titles.

Get your children to school on time, properly dressed, and prepared with what they need for the day.

Do not express disrespect for the teacher or administrator to your children or in front of your children.

Let your children know that in the school the faculty and administration are in charge.

If there is a disagreement or an issue between your child and a teacher or an administrator, address it privately with the appropriate school representatives.

Try This at Home

At many churches that hold more than one service on Sundays, one is typically more family friendly—usually it is the early service. Getting young children ready for church on Sunday mornings can be frantic, and what gets left behind is something to keep them occupied, which is why you see so many mothers digging through their purses looking for pen and paper on which her child can draw. Keep some things that are appropriate for church in your car: a sketch pad, a coloring book, and a plastic bag full of crayons (not a pencil box, which can get very loud when kids rattle it around looking for a particular color), a workbook, or a favorite picture book. These also come in handy at restaurants that do not distribute kiddie diversions.

Some Good Advice

Everyone is busy, pressed for time, under-helped, and overwhelmed. But make time—somehow, somewhere—to volunteer at your child's school. There are countless opportunities, from weekly tutoring sessions to helping in the office or school clinic once every two weeks to chaperoning field trips a few times a year. It is the best way to get to know the teachers and school administration, as well as your child's friends and other parents. If school administrators and teachers can connect your face with your son's face, and know you are actively engaged and supportive of their work, it will without doubt benefit your child. Even one hour a month makes a difference. Your child will be proud to have you there, so enjoy it while you can. Once he enters adolescence, if you dare to show up at his school, he will act as though he has never seen you before in his life.

Chapter Nineteen

BULLIES AND BULLYING

From the time my children were babies until they began school, I was in a weekly playgroup with six mothers and about a dozen children. All the mothers either worked from home or worked part-time, and we were fortunate to have flexible schedules that permitted us to have that special time with our kids and each other.

From early spring until the first freeze, we met every Thursday morning at a child-friendly park with a paved walking track, a small playground, a large sandy area, plenty of grass, and picnic tables. We began arriving around 9:30 a.m., unloading our cars of kids and supplies, toting picnic lunches, diaper bags, blankets, small riding toys, balls, and buckets and shovels for the sand. The kids played (mostly) happily together while the mothers—forming a perimeter around the playground—yakked away until lunchtime. After eating, picking up, packing up, and reloading the cars, we sped home to get the kids to bed for afternoon naps.

Other than some rare and relatively minor squabbles over swings or which sibling got to use the new scooter, those mornings were pretty easygoing, and under six pair of mothers' eyes (not including the ones in the backs of our heads), our children learned and practiced the basics of fair play.

There was one exception and, though rare, it certainly darkened even the sunniest day. A woman we had all known before having children continued to work full time outside the home after her son was born—her only child was cared for by a nanny. About every two months she took a morning off work and with the nanny in tow, she joined us at the park.

From the moment her car pulled up and her son jumped out, our kids were on guard. The boy, who was larger and heavier than the other children, wasted no time asserting himself. Running determinedly through sand castles and moats, pushing to the front of one line at the slide, then another at the water fountain, grabbing toys that caught his fancy for a moment, then throwing them down, hijacking a three-wheeler and racing off, leaving the previous rider in tears—the kid was an aspiring Attila the Hun. All the while, his mother chattered away, blissfully ignorant of the havoc her little darling was wreaking. If one of us pointed anything out, her answer was, "Oh, relax! Boys will be boys."

Yes, they will. But boys should never be permitted to be bullies, and that is exactly what that boy was. His presence inevitably shortened our stay, hurrying our kids off the playground and racing through lunch, eager to get away from the little heathen.

Though I am certain the other moms talked to their kids privately about his behavior—just as I did—we should have been more assertive in letting his mother know what he did was unacceptable.

Bullying has always been frowned upon, but up until the last twenty years or so, bullying and being bullied was considered just one of those childhood things, a rite of passage everyone would eventually outgrow.

But we know differently now. The American Academy of Child and Adolescent Psychiatry estimates up to half of all children are bullied at some point to some degree during their school years.

Boy bullying tends to be more physical than girl bullying, which leans toward being relational and exclusionary. Both types can cause serious harm and have lasting effects.

There are three general types of bullying to be watchful for: physical, verbal, and cyber. Talk to your son about all three of these. Be clear and firm in stating that engaging in any of them will not be tolerated. Be equally firm in stating that if he is subjected to any of these forms of bullying, he must come to you so you can help him.

Schools should be active in identifying children

who may be subjects of bullying as well as the perpetrators. School-wide awareness and bullying prevention programs should be initiated as early as kindergarten; ask your son's teacher or principal if one is in place at your school. If not, volunteer to find one. If your school declines to address the issue, look for seminars presented through a local YMCA, community center, or scouting group. There are many books on the topic, and a wealth of information on the Internet.

As helpful as it can be for communication and research, the Internet is also where some of the most vicious and harmful bullying is born, festers, and spreads. If your son is the subject of a cyber attack, you and he will likely need professional technical assistance to bring it to an end.

You Know You Are Raising a Gentleman If . . .

He does not push other children down, and he apologizes if he does so accidentally.

He does not throw toys, sticks, rocks, or sand, and he never knocks down something another boy has built.

He does not snatch toys from other children.

He waits his turn in line for the slide, climbing wall, or water fountain.

He does not form clubs with the purpose of excluding other children.

He does not call someone names intended to hurt their feelings or call attention to something the person is sensitive about, such as their size or a speech impediment.

When he can, he comes to the defense of a classmate who is being teased or harassed by bullies. If it is not safe for him to do so, he lets an adult know that another child needs help.

He does not join social media groups formed with the intention of harassing or ostracizing anyone.

He does not send mean or threatening messages through texting or social networking, or send or post photos that would hurt or embarrass anyone.

He does not give out his social network passwords, even to his best friend, and always logs out of whatever computer he is using.

Parent Pointers

Talk to your son about what bullying is and how harmful it can be to a child who is bullied.

If you see your son hurting another child, or you suspect he is being deliberately mean to another child, address it calmly, but immediately and purposefully. Don't stop talking about it until you are sure he understands that what he is doing is wrong and unacceptable.

Explain to your son that if he is being bullied in any way, he should tell you so you can help him handle it.

Tell your son that if he sees another child being bullied, or suspects another child is being abused in some way, he should share that privately with an adult.

Educate yourself about bullying—its impact, how to recognize the signs your son or another child is being bullied, and how to respond.

If your son's school does not offer bullying awareness for students, urge them to do so, beginning with the basics in kindergarten and continuing at every grade level with developmental appropriateness.

If your son has been bullied at school, talk to the teacher and administration and make them aware of the problem. Ask that they speak also to anyone who has contact with the bully and the child being bullied, such as librarians, cafeteria workers, and playground supervisors. If that doesn't end the bullying, request a meeting at the school with the perpetrator's parents, teachers, and administration.

Be clear of the potential devastating effects of cyber bullying, as well as the legal consequences.

Make sure your son knows that if he has been subjected to any type of cyber attack, he should not respond or engage, as that will only escalate the attack. He should not delete whatever has been sent or posted, but come to his parents immediately and show them, even if what has been posted is embarrassing to him.

Try This at Home

If you suspect or know for certain that your son has been picked on, or if he is very small for his age—which might cause bigger boys to pick on him—consider enrolling him in a self-defense or martial arts class. While he should never be encouraged or advised to hit back, learning the discipline and focus required of martial arts such as karate, tae kwon do, judo, aikido, or jujitsu will help him develop self-confidence and body awareness.

Some Good Advice

Despite your best efforts to establish open communication with your son, he may be afraid of being labeled a tattletale and not tell you that he is being bullied. Be alert for some telltale signs. Does he seem to have very few friends? Does he have unexplained bruises, cuts, or any other injuries? Have his clothes been torn or are some of his possessions missing? Have his grades dropped? Does he dread going to school? Pay attention to nonverbal signals your son is sending you, and have a private, calm, reassuring talk with him. Chances are, if it is happening, he wants to tell you but doesn't know how.

Chapter Twenty

GOOD SPORTSMANSHIP

S ome of the most blatant exhibitions of bad
sportsmanship ever witnessed have taken place
not in professional sports stadiums and arenas, but
at children's soccer, basketball, hockey, softball, and
baseball games. Even worse, the ugly outbursts have
come, not from children, but from their parents. The
most horrifying incidents make the national news, but
even levelheaded parents can get carried away in the
heat of the moment and do discourteous things like
loudly berating an umpire for what they believe to be a
bad call, or cursing at an opposing coach.

When my son was seven years old, he was playing
a game in a YMCA basketball league on one side of
the gym while two other teams played on the other
side. My son's team finished early, and we stayed to
watch the other match. We saw more than basketball.
Immediately following the game, the mother of a
player on the losing side walked briskly across the

court to the coach of the winning team, slapped him hard across the face, grabbed her son's hand, and stomped out the door. You could have heard a feather drop in that gymnasium; everyone—the coach, players, parents, referees—was stunned into utter silence and her own child was mortified. We knew her to be a good mother and a devoted volunteer at the school. She was one of us, and it made us all feel a little bit ashamed.

Sadly, the boy withdrew from the league; whether it was his choice or his mother's we don't know. The upside of this was that it challenged every parent there to take a good look in the mirror and reinforce the lessons of good sportsmanship.

Long before your son sets foot on a soccer field or basketball court, he will have many opportunities to learn good sportsmanship. When playing board games, for instance, your son will no doubt be disappointed if he is sent to jail without passing go or sent back to Gumdrop Village two spaces from the summit of Candy Mountain. When your son experiences such a setback, do not be tempted to allow him to draw again for a better card. The only way a child can learn to be a good loser is by losing, seeing that it is not the end of the world and that earned success is all that much sweeter.

My son is an excellent athlete, but it pains me to say being a good loser has come with some difficulty. His superior motor skills, competitiveness, and perfectionism combine for some potentially volatile moments on the playing field. It has not been a lesson easily learned. It has required repeated drills, reminders, positive reinforcement, and tough love, including pulling him out of a game or off a field when his conduct warrants it. But, good sportsmanship is an essential character tool for every young man, and for those who are athletically inclined, it is just as important as being able to pitch a baseball or score a goal.

Once your son is signed up for a team sport, you relinquish authority to the coach when he is on the field or court. When playing in a team sport, a young gentleman acknowledges his coach's authority and role and relinquishes his individual aspirations for the common goal of the team.

A coach is charged with teaching the rules of the game and good manners during the competition. Besides a strong pitching arm or quick feet, there are more intangible tools a young man brings to the game. A young gentleman has a positive, generous attitude, always aware that a team sport requires teamwork. He doesn't hog the ball but passes to a teammate who is in a better position to score. If he misses the shot or strikes out, he can show that he is disappointed, but he does not stomp his feet, kick the goal post, throw the bat, or toss his batting helmet.

In some sports, unseemly shows of temper are enough to get a player ejected from the game. I have always found the penalty box in hockey to be a good compromise. In the heat of competition misconduct will occur, but making the offending player sit in the penalty box allows for different degrees of punishment: two minutes, five minutes, or more, depending on the infraction. We have occasionally employed the penalty box concept at home for behavioral missteps.

A young gentleman doesn't question or argue the decisions of the coach or the call of the umpire or referee, nor does he roll his eyes or make disrespectful faces. When it is time for the sides to change, or play to resume, he hustles and does not hold up the game. A young gentleman does not offer excuses for a mistake or bad play—"the sun was in my eyes," "I had a crick in my neck"—but apologizes to his teammates for any lapse that may have hurt the team. A young gentleman accepts the apology from a teammate who made an error, and he does not make fun of an error by a member of the opposing team.

In most children's sports, after the game is concluded, both sides line up and shake hands—or exchange hand slaps—with the opposing players. A young gentleman participates in this ritual with sincerity, without grumpiness or boasting, remembering that being a gracious winner is as important as being a good loser.

The rules of good sportsmanship apply to any competition, whether it is organized sports or playground kickball, a casual race across the swimming pool or a crucial swim meet, or a friendly game of Monopoly. Be fair, be generous, be accommodating, be flexible, and be willing to compromise. Without those principles of play, no one wins.

You Know You Are Raising a Gentleman If . . .

He does not gloat over a win or sulk over a loss.

He does not accuse another player of cheating, even if he knows it to be true.

He knows the rules of play but is willing to consult the rule book if a call or play is in dispute.

He yields to the authority of his coach and referees.

He does not cross the line between aggressive play and assault.

He does not deliberately harm, push, pull, or elbow another player, despite what he may see on television.

He stays engaged in the game, on the field, or from the bench.

He does not make fun of another player's mistakes, even players on opposing teams.

He commends the efforts of a teammate, even if that effort fails.

He acts as a booster for his teammates.

He congratulates the winner if he loses and thanks the losers for a good game if he wins.

When his team is the visitor, he respects the fact that he is a guest in the opposing team's home.

Parent Pointers

Do not "let" your children win a game.

Remind your son that games are meant to be fun, and if his conduct is making it less so, he cannot play.

Remind your son to include everyone who wants to play in the game, even if the child's ability is not commensurate with his teammates.

Help your son learn the rules and peculiar courtesies of the game or sport in which he has chosen to participate.

Yield to the authority of the coaches and referees. If they need your advice, opinion, or help, they will ask.

Do not do anything to embarrass your child, whether that be cursing at the umpire or calling your son by a private family nickname when he comes to bat.

Resist the urge—this is particularly true for mothers—to run onto the field or court and check your child's injury.

Resist the urge—this is particularly true for

fathers—to usurp the coach's game plan or question his or her decisions.

If you have a question about a decision or your son's playing time, consult privately, calmly, and nonconfrontationally with the coach after the game or the day after.

Never berate, yell, or curse at your son, his teammates, opposing players, opposing coaches, opposing parents, or officials.

Act as every child's booster, not just your own. This includes applauding a particularly exceptional play by an opposing player.

Congratulate the winners if you lose; commend the losers for a good effort if you win.

Try This at Home

I abhor the playground practice of "picking" teams. One by one, the best players are chosen, as the lesser ones shrink slowly, inch by inch, into the earth, until finally, only two remain, thoroughly humiliated, dreading the next selection that will reveal which of the two is the least wanted child. I am not an advocate of finding every inane opportunity to boost a child's self-esteem, but this practice destroys a boy's confidence. Parents, teachers, and PE instructors should use a less discriminatory and very simple method. Place the children in a straight line and have them count off one, two, three, four; one, two, three, four. All the ones and threes go on one side, and all the twos and fours go on the other. Allowing children to "pick" the best players first in order to stack a team belies the lesson that it's just a game.

Some Good Advice

Often, a young boy is so disappointed in his play, or his failure, or the result of the game that he will melt down in tears. Competitions—ball games or spelling bees—are intense, and emotions are close to the surface. Crying is a better reaction to disappointment than anger or violence, and it is not a release permitted only to girls. Let a boy work through it and pull himself together; it only takes a minute. A good coach will pull the boy aside for a moment, remind him that it is only a game, and say something to boost his self-confidence. As instinctual as it is for a parent to want to comfort his or her son, do not call attention to his crying by trying to console him or by hissing at him to stop being a crybaby. A ten-year-old chess whiz or eight-year-old swimming star is still a child, not a miniature adult.

Chapter Twenty-one

WRITTEN
CORRESPONDENCE

S omewhere—in a special box, in his baby book,
in the bottom of a drawer—are tucked away
your child's first scribbled communications. Short and
sweet, embellished with a heart or a flower or a stick
figure, they are timelessly endearing in their earnest
simplicity.

Written correspondence is one of the greatest,
most enduring and priceless gifts we can offer one
another. There is a solid argument to be made for
the marvels of e-mail and how well it facilitates easy
and frequent communication among people who
haven't put pen to paper in years. Yet there is still
something very special about finding—amid the
bills, advertisements, solicitations, appointment
reminders, and credit card offers—a handwritten
note or letter from an old friend, a faraway relative,
or a favorite child.

According to standard rules of etiquette, there are three types of letters that should always be handwritten (unless a disability prevents it): notes of condolence, replies to formal invitations, and thank-you notes.

Children will have rare occasion to write condolence notes or reply to formal invitations, but many more opportunities to write thank-you notes. Getting children into the habit of writing thank-you notes at an early age, even before they are able to write a real word, is a good policy that will help them down the road. Make it fun for them, and make good use of their imagination. When my children were toddlers we used finger paints to put their handprints on sheets of paper, then they wrote their names as best they could. I would add a short note of my own. Later we graduated to drawing pictures of the gifts they had received, and finally worked our way up to writing. Stationery companies make preprinted fill-in-the-blank thank-you cards for children. "Dear _____, Thank you for the _____. I love it! _____." Frankly, I'd prefer a paper towel with a Kool-Aid stain and a crayoned scrawl, but something is better than nothing.

It is important that your son understand that when someone is thoughtful enough to remember him with a gift, that gesture must be acknowledged in a personal and prompt fashion (though late is better than never at all).

A child's thank-you notes can be written on almost anything at all, but providing a box of note cards that he chooses himself seems to make the endeavor more bearable. Children's stationery is usually ruled, which is helpful, and can be imprinted with your child's first name. More than any other type of letter, thank-you notes can be written in a conversational style, which is the way most children naturally write anyway. A young gentleman begins his thank-you note with the appropriate salutation: "Dear Grandma," "Dear Aunt Donnie," or "Dear Andrew." If the gift is from a family, he writes, "Dear Shaws" or "Dear Shaw Family."

He acknowledges the specific gift with a brief note of what makes it special: "Thank you for the bat. I hit at least a hundred balls with it at the park yesterday!" or "Thank you for the Harry Potter book. Those are my favorites and I am already on chapter four."

Boys' birthday parties are typically frenetic affairs, but it is important that, when a young gentleman opens his presents, he keeps the accompanying card with the present or opens them at a slow pace, allowing someone to keep a list of the gifts and the givers. It is rude to race through a pile of presents.

If he received cash, he makes some mention of how he has used it, or how he intends to. "Thank you for the check for $25. I used it to get a new soccer ball." Or, "Thank you for the check for my birthday. My mom is taking me to the store this weekend to get a chessboard." In the case of a gift certificate, he can write, "Thank you for the gift certificate to the Apple store. They have the coolest things and I can't wait to go!"

If the gift is from a friend who came to a birthday party, he might add, "Thanks for coming to my party. It was fun." If the gift is from a relative who lives far away, he might say, "It was nice of you to remember me on my birthday. I wish you could have been here."

In closing, he can simply say to a friend, "Thanks again. Harry." To a relative he could say, "Thank you again. Love, Harry." To someone far away, he can write, "I hope to see you soon. Harry."

A young gentleman, who has legible handwriting, addresses the envelopes, then seals and stamps them, saving his parent the trouble.

When a boy is nine or ten years old, he is old enough to write and send the invitations to his own birthday parties. These can be preprinted or designed by the young man on a computer.

You Know You Are Raising a Gentleman If . . .

He handwrites his thank-you notes.

He acknowledges a gift with a thank-you note as promptly as possible.

He includes a reference to the specific gift in the thank-you note. He does not say, "Thank you for the birthday present."

He sends a thank-you note if he has been someone's guest on a special vacation or outing.

He understands privacy issues when it comes to mail, and never opens or reads another person's mail.

Parent Pointers

Handwrite your thank-you notes in a timely and personal fashion.

Get your son in the habit of writing thank-you notes as young as possible. If he can pick up a crayon, he is ready.

Allow your son to choose a box of his own note cards and give him a supply of return address labels and stamps.

If he is too young to do so, address the envelopes
for him as soon as he completes the letter.

Take your son to the post office or mailbox to
drop his letters.

Try This at Home

Another year, another birthday party, another dozen
toys to add to the pile in his bedroom or playroom.
When a major gift-receiving occasion occurs, take the
opportunity to cull from his collection those toys or
gadgets he no longer plays with or uses. The toys he
discards do not need to equal the number of gifts he
has received, but should be significant. If the toys he
is eliminating are in good condition, take them to a
family shelter or day care center for indigent families.

Some Good Advice

My son, as grateful as he is for gifts and kindnesses,
balks when I tell him he needs to write his thank-you
notes. He would much rather be outside playing ball.
After I have nagged him a few days and he still hasn't
sat down at the kitchen table to attend to the task, I
tell him that if it would save him the time, I would be
happy to spare him the trouble of writing notes and
either send his gifts back, or donate them to a local
children's home. That always does the trick.

Chapter Twenty-two

GIVING AND RECEIVING

E very December since I was seven years old, I have hung the same special ornament on my Christmas tree. It began its holiday decorating career as a red Christmas ball, onto which had been glued a pair of blue eyes, a nose, and a bow-shaped mouth. A little felt Santa hat with a piece of holly was perched on top, and from under the hat hung two braids of yellow yarn.

Until I left home it was stored with all our other family ornaments, but it was never unwrapped or hung up by anyone but me. When I left at nineteen to move to New York City, along with my clothes, furniture, family photos, books, records, and diaries, I took the ornament, wrapped in tissue paper in a small box. That first lonely Christmas there in my tiny studio apartment, it was the only decoration I placed on my tabletop tree. My collection of ornaments grows larger every year, but that one started it all. It moved with me to six different apartments in New York and then to Nashville and three different homes there. Over the years she cracked from one side to another, and I taped her back up again. Then she lost one eye, then her nose, and finally, the ball itself became so shattered, it was not repairable. The only parts that now remain on the hook are the hat and the braids, and they are looking pretty shabby too. A couple of years ago, my children were laughing at the raggedy thing and asked me why I didn't just throw it away. Here is what I told them:

When I was seven years old, my Brownie troop celebrated Christmas by making stockings of personal items and taking them to a nursing home for senior citizens, where we sang Christmas carols and had punch and cookies. Afterward, we returned to the church where we held our meetings for the eagerly awaited gift exchange. Every Brownie had been told to bring a gift with a three-dollar limit. The wrapped presents were put in a pile, and one by one, we chose one and opened it. I was the last to pick, and watched as the other Brownies opened boxes of colored pencils, a game, or small pieces of jewelry. Finally, it was my turn and I opened the last small box. Inside was the ornament. I was sorely disappointed at such a useless gift, and if the look on my face wasn't obvious enough,

I saw fit to say aloud, "What is this?" with a tone of utter dismay.

As soon as the words left my mouth, I knew I had done something really, really wrong. The little girl who had contributed the ornament—which she had made with her mother—burst into tears. My ignominy was heightened by the fact that my mother was the Brownie leader. She was astonished at this behavior from her very own child, and she snatched me up from my seat so quickly I thought she would pull my arm out of its socket. She marched me out of the room and into the hall, where she told me in no uncertain terms that she had never been so embarrassed or so ashamed of me. Of course I had to apologize to my fellow Brownie, and to her mother when she came to pick up her daughter. For the rest of the year, that Brownie didn't speak to me, and I didn't blame her a bit. The odd thing was that my reaction was completely out of character for me, heretofore a warmhearted and sweet-natured child, and to this day I still have no idea what could have come over me to treat another person so cruelly.

When we got home, I was sent to my room, where I flung myself on my bed and cried and cried. Finally, my mother came in and, now somewhat calmed down, gave me a lecture on kindness, decency, consideration, and respect, but it wasn't really necessary. The little girl's hurt face that afternoon spoke volumes and had already taught me all I needed to know. I wrote her a thank-you note, with another apology, then hung the ornament on our tree.

For the first several years after that Christmas, every time I hung the ornament I was again overwhelmed with shame and regret at my actions that day. Over time, the sting has lessened, but I have never once hung that ornament without its attendant reminder of my thoughtless action.

I didn't relish sharing that story with my children, but I hope it accomplished a few things. They saw that even their mother, still perfect in every way to a seven- and eight-year-old, had once (if only it were just once) done something very wrong, and that when we do something wrong, we must make amends. They also learned that receiving graciously is a gift you return to the giver, and that causing someone unnecessary hurt will cause you the far greater pain. My mother had forgotten the entire incident until I brought it up a few years ago. I'll bet that the little girl hasn't given it a thought in years and years. But because of what my parents had already taught me about how to treat others, and thanks to a tiny Santa hat that hangs on a crooked hook, I will never forget that afternoon. As painful as it is, I am grateful for the reminder.

More than anything else, good parents give their children daily examples of respect, kindness, consideration, honor, generosity, empathy, charity, compassion, and grace. These are the most profound gifts you can bestow upon your children and the ones that will last their lifetime.

ABOUT THE AUTHOR

KAY WEST has been a professional writer in Nashville, TN for 30 years. She was restaurant critic for the *Nashville Scene* for 15 years and remains a contributing feature writer. She is Nashville stringer for People. She has written four books, including *How to Raise a Lady* and *How to Raise a Gentleman*, and co-authored *Dani's Story: A Journey From Neglect to Love*. She has raised a well-mannered daughter and a well-mannered son and is an avid baseball fan.

INDEX

D

J

K

L

911 calls, 117, 122
nose, picking, 88

O

obscene phone calls, 122
offering seat to others, 80, 83
office, bringing child to, 25–26
opera, 73
opinions, accepting differences, 109

P

pants, sagging, 96
parental control software, 126–127
parents
    child's sharing time with, 24–25
    drive for son's success, ix–x
    enforcement of behavior on airplane, 77
    and errands, 28
    handling temper tantrums, 101–108
    poor sportsmanship from, 157–158
parked car, child alone in, 29
participation, in church services, 146
parties, delayed arrival, 53
party manners, 47–55
passing food at mealtime, 58
passing gas, 86, 89, 91
passing judgment, on spiritual or political beliefs, 114
performances
    coughing during, 72
    enjoyment of, 66
    seating for, 67
    talking during, 67
photographs, 93–94
physical bullying, 151
physical handicaps, 134
picking noses, 88
picking teams, 163–164
playdates, 31–33
    invitations for, 34
    parent pointers, 35
playgrounds, 33

R